Medicine and Society

Medicine and Society

Clinical Decisions and Societal Values

Cornell University Medical College
Third Conference on Health Policy

edited by
Eli Ginzberg

WESTVIEW PRESS
BOULDER AND LONDON

Conservation of Human Resources Studies in Health Policy

Published in 1987 in the United States of America by Westview Press, Inc.; Frederick A. Praeger, Publisher; 5500 Central Avenue, Boulder, Colorado 80301

Library of Congress Catalog Card Number: 87-50603
ISBN: 0-8133-0574-8

Composition for this book originated with conversion of the author's computer tapes or word-processor disks.
This book was produced without formal editing by the publisher.

Printed and bound in the United States of America

∞ The paper used in this publication meets the requirements of the American National Standard for Permanence of Paper for Printed Library Materials Z39.48-1984.

6 5 4 3 2 1

Contents

List of Tables and Figures vii
Foreword, Thomas H. Meikle, Jr. ix

1 The Setting, *Eli Ginzberg* 1

2 A Twentieth Century Retrospective, *Robert H. Ebert* 7

3 Allocating Health Care Resources: How Can We Ensure Access to Essential Care?
Albert L. Siu and Robert H. Brook 20

4 Alternative Treatments and Outcomes for Patients with Cardiovascular Diseases, *J. G. G. Ledingham* 34

5 A Catastrophic Disease Perspective on Organ Transplantation, *Roger W. Evans* 61

6 Aging Reconsidered: Emerging Research and Policy Issues,
John W. Rowe and Robert H. Binstock 96

7 The New Genetics and the Future Practice of Medicine,
Leon E. Rosenberg 114

8 Themes and Policies, *Eli Ginzberg* 132

About the Contributors 141
Cornell University Medical College Third Conference on Health Policy 143
Index 145

Tables and Figures

Tables

4.1	Data from the Australian National Blood Pressure Study	37
4.2	Data from CASS	48
4.3	Treatment of myocardial infarction by patient category and type of hospital, Denmark, 1986	54
4.4	Treatment of acute myocardial infarction by type of hospital, Denmark, 1986	55
5.1	Need for organ transplant procedures in the United States	64
5.2	Estimates of the number of organ donors in the United States, 1980–1985	65
5.3	Patient groups and measures relevant to cost-effectiveness of organ transplantation	69
5.4	Estimated charges associated with various solid organ transplant procedures	70
5.5	Reimbursement made by the Medicare program for services provided to ESRD patients through June 30, 1986	72
5.6	Number of kidney transplants performed by year, 1973–1985	73
5.7	Transplant survival rates	74
5.8	Summary of quality of life scores for heart transplant, kidney transplant, and kidney dialysis patients	75
5.9	Definition of catastrophic medical expenses: Key elements and perspectives	77
5.10	Ten leading causes of death in the United States, 1985	81
5.11	Estimated risk of death to an individual from various human-caused and natural accidents	84

Figures

4.1	Coronary heart disease mortality, males and females, aged 35–74, selected countries, 1968–1982	42
4.2	Average percentage change in mortality from ischemic	

disease, males and females, aged 40–69, selected countries, 1968–1979 44
4.3 European Coronary Surgery Study and Coronary Artery Surgery Study 47
4.4 Correlation between the attack rate of acute myocardial infarction and the death rate, males and females, aged 55–64 49
5.1 Conceptualization of the costs of disease and illness 79

Foreword

Medicine and Society: Clinical Decisions and Societal Values reflects the theme of the Cornell University Medical College Third Conference on Health Policy, a series made possible by an anonymous gift of $50 million to the Medical College that specified the development of a program on health policy as part of that gift. The intent of the conferences has been to probe in depth major issues that have the potential of altering in fundamental ways the structure of medicine—how it is practiced, what it does, and whom it benefits.

The first conference, held in 1985 (*The U.S. Health Care System: A Look to the 1990s*), considered how the health care delivery system was changing in the 1980s and how these changes in an increasingly market-oriented environment threatened access by the poor to health care. The conference that followed in 1986 focused on two conflicting developments: the continuing large increase in the number of physicians in proportion to the population and the development of new, managed health care systems and their influence on medical practice (*From Physician Shortage to Patient Shortage: The Uncertain Future of Medical Practice*). This year's conference focuses on new frontiers of clinical medicine and the dilemmas they pose for society and the profession.

As before, the backbone of the conference consisted of six specially prepared papers that provided the points of departure for the two-day discussion. They are contained in this volume together with an introductory chapter and summary of the proceedings written by the conference chairman.

The Third Conference builds upon the themes of its predecessors. Its focus is derived from those discussions that identified as a fundamental issue the translation of societal values into health care objectives and the formulation of mechanisms by which these objectives could guide the process of making clinical decisions. That is, how should society or the individual physician make clinical decisions regarding individual patient care that are consistent with societal goals and values? The authors of the basic papers seem to agree on several principles: First, all persons, regardless of individual resources, should be provided access to something that is defined as "essential health care"; second, care should be demonstrably effective and beneficial; and third, care should be delivered efficiently in a cost-effective manner.

Although it is not my intent to specify the agenda or the outcome of the conference, I would hope that we would seek operational definitions as to what constitutes "essential," "effective," and "efficient" health care. How does one define essential medical care and is it, in fact, an entitled right or should it be? Or, are the terms congruent? Is essential medical care principally oriented to prolonging life or to enhancing specific aspects or qualities of life? And is essential care the same for the young and the elderly? How will an aging population and new technology affect the definition of essential medical care?

Turning to our second principle, what is clinically effective and beneficial medical care? Do few medical treatments actually have clear-cut outcomes? How difficult is it to determine the effectiveness of medical treatment? What would be the impact on medical education, medical care, and the profession, if prescribed therapeutic protocols became usual practice? And would such an approach to treatment yield significant financial savings? Would the elimination of ineffective therapeutic procedures and regimens produce real savings in health care costs? And again, what would be the effects of new medical technology and the aging of the population on the definition of effective, beneficial medical care?

Finally, how does one define cost-efficient medical care? Is there validity to the concept of an arbitrary cap on per capita health care expenditures or on the percentage of GNP devoted to health care? Or a defensible method of estimating it? Should health care resources be allocated differently to different age groups? Does prevention of illness prolong life and ultimately result in increased health care outlays? And will new technology significantly reduce or increase total health care costs over the long term?

Issues such as these are the legacy of the extraordinary progress that medicine has made in the past half century. Our capacity and willingness to deal with these issues will determine the willingness of the society to support a comparable level of progress in the future.

The partnership of Cornell University Medical College and the Conservation of Human Resources has been especially successful as a joint effort to examine issues that reflect both societal and medical concerns. The credit for the success of these conferences goes to Eli Ginzberg. As in previous years, I would like to acknowledge his expert chairmanship and great skill in conceptualizing and planning these conferences. The participation and support of Associate Dean Michael J. Sniffen, who also serves as executive director of the Cornell Health Policy Program, has been invaluable. Theda Jensen of the associate dean's office handled the many details of assembling and accommodating our out-of-town participants.

Conservation of Human Resources staff members Miriam Ostow, Howard Berliner, and, most particularly, Penny Peace, oversaw and coordinated the numerous steps in the development of the conference. I am again indebted to Ruth Szold Ginzberg for her sensitive editing of the papers for publication.

Thomas H. Meikle, Jr., M.D.
The Stephen and Suzanne Weiss Dean
Cornell University Medical College

1

The Setting

Eli Ginzberg

The purpose of this introduction is to identify the principal themes that have been addressed by the contributors to this volume and to help the reader discern the linkages among them. Each of the chapters was written as a background paper for a conference on *Medicine and Society: Clinical Decisions and Societal Values* and provided the point of departure for two days of lively, fruitful discussion among a group of academic physicians, social scientists, and government officials.

In Chapter 2, *A Twentieth Century Retrospective,* Dr. Robert Ebert has conceptualized the principal forces that transformed American medicine in the twentieth century. He identifies four: the dominant role of science and technology in altering the ecology of disease; the profound impact that scientific and technological advances have had on the entire matrix of the medical enterprise; the interactive effects of changes in medicine and in the sociopolitical framework of the larger society in which it is embedded; and dangers to the individual and society created by the public's unrealistic expectations of the potential of scientific medicine.

After assessing the contribution of each to altering the structure and functioning of our health care system, Dr. Ebert raises a number of policy implications in which he seeks to tie the past to the future. The past, he notes, will prove simpler than the future, partly because the advances in health care have altered so many fundamental aspects of contemporary society, not the least being the much larger proportion of the population that lives to old age. This in turn evokes a large number of ethical issues, including such basic questions as the considerations that should govern efforts to prolong life or speed death.

Drawing on his own long and distinguished career as a medical educator, Dr. Ebert believes that substantial changes are called for in the preparation of tomorrow's physicians at both the undergraduate and the graduate level, in particular a better articulation of the two. Such changes could reduce the length and cost of medical education, increase its effectiveness, and produce a better mix of primary care physicians and specialists.

In his concluding section, Dr. Ebert also raises some interesting questions about the likely shifts that will occur in the relations between physicians and hospitals, the various systems of health care delivery, and the boundaries of medicine in a society in which the demarcation between medicine and other realms is often difficult to discern and is subject to change as societal values change.

Chapter 3, *Allocating Health Care Resources: How Can We Ensure Access to Essential Care?*, by Drs. Siu and Brook of the University of California, Los Angeles and the Rand Corporation, addresses head-on one of the most critical issues to have preoccupied the U.S. health care sector since the late 1950s–early 1960s when public concern was focused on the economic barriers that were blocking access to the system for a large number of the elderly and the poor. For a brief period after the passage of Medicare and Medicaid in 1965 it appeared that this shortfall would be corrected; since the early 1980s, however, as Congress and the corporate sector have faced increasing financial pressures, economic barriers to care have again mounted.

Siu and Brook pose the question: Are the resources available to the U.S. health care system in 1987 (over half a trillion dollars) sufficient to assure access to "essential care" for all persons irrespective of their ability to pay? A subsidiary consideration that the authors address is: Can effective care for all be assured without resorting to "rationing"? This has been the response of the National Health Service in the United Kingdom and the health systems of various other countries when confronted with a substantial gap between the demand (need) for care and the resources available.

Siu and Brook develop their answer in stages. They first argue that there is considerable evidence to indicate that many health care services currently provided, including hospitalization and high-cost surgery, are not justified and are, in fact, often contraindicated because they are potentially harmful to the patient. Further, many costly services have, at best, an equivocal cost/benefit ratio, with the value of their outcome problematic. Accordingly, the authors conclude that if the expenditures for all of the former and some of the latter could be recaptured and the resources directed to expanding medical care for needy patients, the current level of expenditures would be more than ample to assure that all persons have access to "essential care."

The authors conclude their presentation by specifying ways to move toward their desired goal. They make a strong plea for the professional leadership, particularly at academic health centers, to take the lead in identifying costly procedures that should be outlawed; they suggest that certain equivocal procedures be performed only at selected institutions under strict protocols and the results submitted to systematic analysis; and they point to audits of physician records as a means of assessing retrospectively the appropriateness of customary diagnostic and therapeutic interventions in order to eliminate unnecessary and costly treatment modalities.

Dr. John Ledingham, Reader in Medicine at Oxford University, was invited to compare the treatment of cardiovascular diseases in Great Britain and other Western European countries with that in the United States. His chapter, *Alternative Treatments and Outcomes for Patients with Cardiovascular Diseases,* addresses the most common pathologies—malignant, severe, and mild hypertension, coronary artery disease, angina pectoris, and acute myocardial infarction.

Dr. Ledingham notes that with respect to some conditions, specifically malignant and severe hypertension, there is a marked conformity in the way in which physicians in all of the advanced countries treat their patients. On the other hand, this is not true in the case of mild hypertension where U.S. physicians are much more likely than their British colleagues to initiate drug treatment. In seeking to explain the difference, the author points to the different readings by the two groups of the conclusions to be extracted from the clinical trials that have been conducted and the preference of British physicians for nonpharmacological interventions.

The British medical profession is less convinced than colleagues in the United States that reducing arterial pressure and lowering blood cholesterol concentrations will necessarily lead to a reduction in mortality from coronary disease. This is not to say that increased pressure and increased cholesterol concentrations are not recognized as risk factors, but only that the British are cautious about inferring that drug therapy to reduce both will result in significant reductions in mortality.

The most striking difference between practice in the United Kingdom and the United States relates to the use of surgical interventions for angina pectoris. The rate of surgery in the United States is currently five times that in Great Britain. Ledingham observes that if resources permitted, the British would like to increase their rate by 50 percent; this would still leave a 3:1 differential in favor of the United States. He further emphasizes that the reduced incidence of coronary disease, not a reduced case fatality rate, is the critical factor.

In reflecting on the differences in treatment modalities between the two countries, Ledingham places heavy weight on such diverse factors as total resource availability, the influence of the prevailing fee-for-service practice mode in the United States, the antitechnologic bias in the United Kingdom, and differing interpretations of the epidemiologic evidence. Clearly, professional (physician) views and preferences combine with societal attitudes and behavior to produce distinctive patterns of clinical practice on each side of the Atlantic.

Nowhere is the confrontation between clinical decisions and societal values sharper than in the area of organ transplantation, particularly as regards kidney, liver, and heart. In his chapter, *A Catastrophic Disease Perspective on Organ Transplantation,* Dr. Roger Evans, who has had unique opportunities to study the steadily increasing body of data and to participate actively in policy formulation, has sought to clarify a large number of conventional misconceptions about the present state of transplantation and likely developments in the period immediately ahead.

He points out that it is incorrect to view transplantation as an open-ended, very costly frontier because of an ever-growing demand/need for organ replacement. Rather, it is the supply of available organs that is the critical factor in assessing utilization of the technology in the present and the near future. In the distant future, if nonhuman organs and/or artificial organs can be used, the supply constraint might be radically reduced, if not totally removed. At the present, the best that one can expect is to enhance the current limited supply through improved collection and distribution systems.

Dr. Evans also explores a series of critical issues connected with the economic and ethical dilemmas that are brought to the surface as a result of the growth of transplantation therapy. He helps the reader to see that such questions as who should have preferred access to the limited supply of organs, who should cover the costs of the transplantation (including preparation and follow-up), how the years of useful life are to be measured, and a variety of related issues are easier to formulate than to resolve. Even if the professionals were able to reach consensus, the public would have to be persuaded.

Drs. Rowe and Binstock, in their chapter, *Aging Reconsidered,* focus on one of the most important transformations that has occurred, the greying of the population, whose impact and influence will be magnified after the turn of the century when the baby-boom generation approaches the age of retirement. The number and proportion of the population that reaches age sixty-five continue to increase and the subgroups of those over seventy-five and over eighty-five are growing particularly rapidly.

The impact of these demographic phenomena on the health care system is underscored by two unequivocal facts—that the population over sixty-five accounts for about three times more health care services than those under sixty-five, and that the demand for services increases with advancing years, particularly the need for nursing home care.

The authors make an important analytic discrimination between the incidence of chronic diseases which are correlated with aging and the phenomena of "normal" and "successful" aging which apply to considerable (and increasing) numbers of people in their sixties, seventies, and eighties who remain substantially free of morbidity.

Based on this discrimination between the sick and the non-sick elderly (although the latter, particularly those older than eighty-five, may have signs of frailty), the authors distill a number of important findings both for physicians who treat the elderly and for the formulation of public policies affecting this population. Their most important observation is to warn against the simple projection into the future of characteristics that have been found among earlier cohorts of the elderly. As they note, future cohorts are likely to reach old age in better physical condition, to be better educated, to face fewer economic problems, and to enjoy other important advantages over those who lived to retirement and longer in earlier decades.

The thrust of the Rowe-Binstock chapter is to alert all readers, whatever their professional background, to the urgency of "reconsidering" aging for the simple reason that current beliefs and attitudes about the elderly are in many respects wrong and, if not corrected, will lead to wrong (ineffective and costly) policies.

Dr. Leon Rosenberg, Dean of the Yale Medical School and a major contributor to the field of medical genetics, is the author of the last of the six specially prepared essays. His title, *The New Genetics: The Future Practice of Medicine,* is indicative of his approach. Rosenberg starts by calling attention to the recency of the field and the unparalleled rapidity of its development. The discovery of recombinant DNA (rDNA), the springboard for the recent spate of dramatic breakthroughs, dates only to 1972.

The author describes the multiple ramifications of this new technology—as a tool for discovery in basic science, as a spur to commercial development (the biotechnology industry), and as a major new tool for clinical medicine. Further, he calls attention to the ethical and moral dilemmas that the new genetics raises because of its present and, even more, potential capacity to determine the birth and survival of normal and handicapped infants.

In the near term Dr. Rosenberg sees the new genetics as effecting a major upheaval in the clinical laboratory where diagnostic evaluation will require the active participation of a consulting geneticist capable of assessing and interpreting the relationships between individual and family group findings.

In addition to the gains on the diagnostic front, important gains are being made through product development and gene therapy. Further advances are found in the areas of disease prevention and health maintenance, especially via genetic epidemiology and prenatal detection.

Nevertheless, Dr. Rosenberg does not overlook important barriers that may slow, if not stop, the potential of this new breakthrough—society's failure to invest adequate (not excessive) sums in ongoing research and development and the prevalence of ignorance and prejudice among large segments of the profession and the public. While conceding that there is ground for caution, he believes that the potential for human benefit far exceeds the dangers that could result from misapplication of the new technology.

What each of the chapters makes clear, and what all six unequivocally confirm, is that medicine and society have always been interactive: Society provides the required resources and enjoys the direct benefits of improved diagnostic and therapeutic interventions while the members of the medical profession occupy key roles as investigators and therapeutic agents. The chapters demonstrate eloquently that the changes occurring in the larger society have a major impact on the needs and demands of the population for new and different medical care; and that advances in medicine can create new opportunities—and also new challenges—for a society that must play an active role in determining the resources that it will devote to improving the quality of its members' lives and extending their life spans. The interface between medicine and society is no longer limited to the halls of the legislature; increasingly it is found in the day-to-day decision-making that takes place at the hospital bedside and in the physician's office.

2

A Twentieth Century Retrospective

Robert H. Ebert

The title of this essay is so broad that it would be easy to become mired in a morass of detail. To avoid that hazard, the discussion to follow is limited to four major themes:

- Science and technology, nurtured by an unprecedented economic development during much of this century, have profoundly altered the ecology of disease.
- This in turn has had an equally profound impact on the matrix of medicine, by which is meant all aspects of medical organization including the way in which medicine is practiced, the structure of the medical care system, the economics of medicine, the nature of medical education, and the characteristics of those entering the profession.
- It is impossible to change the matrix of medicine without changing other aspects of national life, and the policy implications of changes in both the past and the future will be discussed.
- The enormous success of scientific medicine has created what at times is an unrealistic faith in its effectiveness and this has led to both denial of risk and to the medicalization of certain social problems including violence, teenage pregnancy, substance abuse, and even the homeless.

Science, Technology, and the Ecology of Disease

The major forces which have led to change during this century have been science and technology nurtured by economic development in a free, or at least a relatively free, enterprise system. Science and technology, in turn, have enhanced economic development. Two aspects of this dynamic relationship have affected the health of Americans: purposeful changes in the environment made to enhance health and a revolution in the science and technology of medicine sparked by the progress of science in other spheres. A nation that enjoys a strong economy can afford those measures that ensure public health, such as the guarantee of clean water, the drainage of swamps that breed disease-carrying mosquitoes, and even the elimination of the pollution that results from industrial activity or the product of that activity such as automobile emissions.

But it is the quantum leap in scientific medicine during the twentieth century and the greatly accelerated rate of change during the second half of the century that are the major topics of this essay. Much of the groundwork for change was laid in the latter part of the nineteenth century with advances in chemistry, bacteriology, pathology, and physiology, but it wasn't until the late 1930s and early 1940s that the major products of earlier discoveries began to emerge in a way destined to alter the ecology of disease. The most dramatic was the discovery of potent yet safe antibiotics, beginning with the introduction of penicillin during World War II and followed by the discovery of chemotherapeutic agents capable of curing tuberculosis. Curiously, these agents, introduced to treat or prevent infections, have had the greatest impact on the ecology of disease even though they are among the least expensive and least complex of the technologies introduced into medical practice during this century. Consider what they have accomplished. Tuberculosis, for practical purposes, has been eliminated as an important disease for most of the U.S. population. While there had been a steady decline in the mortality and morbidity rates decades before the introduction of modern chemotherapy, tuberculosis remained a serious disease for those with clinical infection; primary infection was so common in this country in the early part of the century that the tuberculin test was considered of little diagnostic value after adolescence since almost everyone would have converted to tuberculin positive as the result of a clinically unimportant primary infection. Today conversion to tuberculin positive is an indicator for treatment.

Syphilis, the great imitator, is no longer a scourge of civilization and syphilitic heart disease and the diseases of the nervous system caused by the spirochaete are rarities in this country today. The heart disease and renal disease so commonly the sequelae of streptococcal infection can be prevented and vaccines against polio, measles, diptheria, rubella, and tetanus have made it possible to close the large communicable disease hospital found in every large city at an earlier time. And, finally, pneumonococcal pneumonia no longer fills hospital wards during the winter months.

This is not to say that infection is a category of disease no longer dreaded, but the ecology of infection has changed, partly because of bacterial resistance to many antibiotics, partly as the result of therapies that affect the immune system, and partly due to the advent of a new epidemic disease—AIDS. As in the years prior to an understanding of the etiology of infection, hospitals have become hazardous places, no longer as the result of ignorance, but because so many infections contracted in hospitals today are caused by organisms resistant to common antibiotics.

The success of organ transplantation depends upon sufficient suppression of the immune response so that transplants are not rejected. But that suppression is not innocuous since it causes the body to become susceptible to organisms that are ordinarily nonpathogenic. Immunosuppressive drugs used to ensure the protection of transplants were discovered in the search for drugs effective against various forms of cancer, and patients receiving cancer chemotherapy are also susceptible to infection with what are ordinarily harmless bacteria.

One of the reasons that AIDS was recognized as a disease that suppressed the immune system even before the cause was known is the earlier experience with immunosuppressive drugs. AIDS reminds us that despite our success in the control of epidemic disease, we are still susceptible to attack by an apparently new pathogenic virus. We also must realize that knowledge about how to prevent the spread of infection is no guarantee that preventive measures will be carried out. On the brighter side, we are reminded of the power of modern science that within a few short years has identified the causative virus and its precise mode of attack on the body's immune system.

There have been remarkable advances in the diagnosis and treatment of the many other diseases that plague mankind, but unfortunately few approaches enable us to prevent or cure these diseases in the way that we can prevent or cure many infections. Most address the consequences of chronic illness and although it is sometimes possible to halt the advance of disease or at least to slow it, treatment is often designed simply to relieve the pain and disability resulting from disease. Advances in obstetrics and neonatology make it possible to avoid some of the complications of dystocia, to anticipate fetal distress, and to preserve life in premature infants who without modern technology would surely die. Yet, we know that human behavior probably plays an even larger part in determining the outcome of pregnancy than all our modern technological appurtenances. If teenage pregnancy could be avoided, at least until the late teens, if all pregnant women would seek early prenatal care, and would avoid drugs, alcohol, and cigarettes during their pregnancies, it is quite likely that more could be done to reduce infant mortality and morbidity than is possible as a consequence of modern science.

There have been remarkable advances in our ability to diagnose with precision the exact location of coronary artery disease and to bypass a diseased vessel thus improving flow to the myocardium. We are able to monitor what is happening electrically to the heart following a myocardial infarction and to halt the abrupt onset of an arrhythmia that may cause sudden death. We are even able to unblock the acutely occluded coronary vessel. But nothing that is done in the coronary care ward or in the operating room can cure the disease. Again, prevention or at least slowing the advance of coronary artery disease is more dependent on diet, exercise, and the avoidance of cigarettes than on the miracles of modern medicine. Fortunately, advances in biomedical knowledge do affect human behavior to a degree. A better understanding of the risk factors affecting cardiovascular disease has caused many people, particularly the better educated, to change their dietary habits, to exercise sensibly, and to avoid cigarettes. Unfortunately, the young, the less well-educated, and the poor are less likely to alter their behavior for health reasons. Children and adolescents today are rarely the victims of acute infections that now can be prevented by vaccination or cured with antibiotics. But medicine can do little to prevent the violence, suicide, auto accidents, and substance abuse that are today's killers of the young.

In addition to a successful U.S. economy for most of this century, what has fueled the advances in the science and technology of medicine, particularly in the second half of the twentieth century? During the early part of the century we were largely dependent on the great renaissance of European biomedical science that began in the nineteenth century and culminated in German medicine prior to World War I. In the brief interval between the world wars, England and France were the preservers of what remained of European scientific medicine, although this country contributed as well, partly by creating strong research environments at academic centers such as the Rockefeller Institute and some large universities and partly by becoming a haven for refugee scientists from Europe. World War II was the turning point, however, that established a framework for the preeminence of American biomedical science after the war. The success of the Manhattan project that established a close working relationship between government and the private sector became the model for the support of biomedical research in the nation's universities, medical schools, and teaching hospitals via the National Institutes of Health (NIH). Congress was convinced that if such a partnership could create the atomic bomb it could also solve the problems of cancer or heart disease, and so money became available for both basic research and the practical applications that derived from that research. The pharmaceutical industry together with manufacturers of medical instruments also realized that their future depended on research and development so they too contributed to the new technology.

The Impact of Science and Technology on the Matrix of Medicine

The advances in the science and technology of medicine changed not only the ecology of disease but the entire matrix of medicine as well, including everything from the relationship between hospitals and doctors to the willingness of government to pay for the fruits of medical invention.

At the beginning of the century the hospital had little to offer in the way of technology, other than surgery, that could not be done at home. While some notable group practices were formed in the early part of the twentieth century and some specialists were clustered in the downtown areas of major cities, the majority of physicians practiced in the neighborhoods they served. As the complexity of medical practice increased, however, and dependency on specialized instrumentation became more imperative, physicians found it convenient to form both formal and informal groups and to locate their offices near the hospital. This trend accelerated rapidly after World War II and was associated with increasing specialization. Less and less time was devoted to home visits as office and hospital practice preempted the physician's working hours.

Further specialization was the inevitable consequence of the explosive expansion of medical knowledge following World War II. While subspecialization was encouraged by the categorical nature of the NIH, it soon became evident that a general internist could not be equally expert in gastroenterology, cardiology, nephrology, and endocrinology. Similarly, no general surgeon could practice urology, orthopedics, abdominal surgery, cardiothoracic surgery, and neurosurgery with the competence of the subspecialist. Inevitably young physicians in training were attracted to these subspecialties. In recent years subspecialization has become even more refined, witness the division of practice among ophthalmologists, some of whom specialize in diseases of the retina, some in corneal disease, and some in treating the manifestations of glaucoma.

In theory the subspecialist is a consultant to other physicians, but in practice he often becomes the primary care provider for individuals with chronic diseases. Thus, the rheumatologist is likely to provide ongoing care for the patient with rheumatoid arthritis just as the cardiologist may become the primary care provider for the patient with coronary artery disease.

In the rapidly changing world of the 1950s and 1960s, the hospital became the major focus of medical practice and the primary teaching hospital became the paradigm, for it was here that subspecialists working in concert with instrument makers and the pharmaceutical industry were revolutionizing the practice of medicine. The specificity, potency, and often the dangerous side effects of new drugs, together with the complexity of new instruments and devices served to enhance the role of the subspecialist. New ways of viewing organs and even blood vessels together with new surgical procedures developed in academic medical centers reinforced the view that subspecialists were needed in community hospitals and that the models of specialty practice and intensive care found in university hospitals should be transplanted to large community hospitals.

Curiously, the formal part of medical education, the medical school, remained relatively unchanged in organization despite the dramatic changes in science, technology, and the ecology of disease. Obviously, the content changed, but the division of time between preclinical and clinical studies remained about the same, and each discipline attempted to transmit as much information as possible during the four years of medical school for fear there would never be another chance. What most educators chose to ignore was that medical education had drastically changed as a consequence of specialization and that most of the clinical education of the physician occurred after graduation during the residency years.

When I was a boy in the 1920s, I was accidentally hit on the head with a steel shotput, resulting in a deep gash in my forehead and a possible concussion. I was hospitalized for three or four days, the wound was sutured, and I was watched to determine if there had been any internal injury to my head. The cost of hospitalization was minimal; no surgical fee was charged since my father was a physician; and although there was no insurance, the out-of-pocket costs were trivial. Contrast that with what would happen today. If hospitalized at all, it would be for no longer than a day; a battery of tests would be done, including a CAT scan. In addition to the hospital bill, fees would be charged by a surgeon, a neurologist (or neurosurgeon), a radiologist, and most of these charges, amounting to many hundreds of dollars, would be covered by insurance. I present this parable to make two points: Changes in medical practice brought about by scientific advance cost a lot of money yet the insured individual feels very little pain from the out-of-pocket expense.

What are the components of medical costs? Drugs and appliances account for 8 percent, physician fees for 19 percent, other professional fees for 9 percent, and hospital costs for 39 percent. The total cost, which in 1985 amounted to $425 billion, continues to escalate because there are developmental costs for new drugs, new instruments, new devices, and new procedures. Even when capital costs are low there is almost always additional technical manpower needed to operate a new instrument, monitor a new drug, or assist in a new procedure. Rarely does one technology completely supplement another; most medical technologies are add-ons to what already exists.

The rapid escalation of medical care costs amounting in recent years (since 1980) to about 12 percent per year has caused those who pay—particularly government and industry—to ask how costs can be controlled without denying the advantages of modern medicine. Several approaches have been tried including prospective payment for hospital care, managed care using primary care physicians as gatekeepers, and care paid for on the basis of capitation—so-called prepaid care. All of these approaches have worked to a degree but none has proven to be a panacea, and short of rationing as in Great Britain, it is unlikely that we will ever reduce what we spend as a percentage of GNP—now approximately 11 percent. Instead we are likely to increase that percentage.

Whatever has or has not been accomplished to control medical care costs, there is little doubt that some profound changes have occurred as a consequence of trying. Because of the high cost of hospital care, more and more procedures including major surgery are being carried out in an ambulatory setting, and the hospital-centered paradigm of the academic health center is no longer the model for the community. Decentralization has been made possible by further advances in medical technology as well as in the technology of computers. In the present competitive environment, attempts at cost control as well as a growing excess of physicians have resulted in different systems which compete with each other for a share of the market. This in turn has led to changes in the characteristics of those who choose a career in medicine, the attitudes of the public toward medicine, even the feelings of physicians about their profession.

People are attracted to the medical profession for a variety of reasons, some because they enjoy working with people, some for altruistic reasons, some because medicine combines science with action, some because of the potential for independence, and some because the profession offers financial security—or at least it did in the past. The mix of interests changes from time to time, and in the 1960s those admitted to medical school were heavily oriented toward what Funkenstein has called the "bioscientific." During the decade of the 1960s medicine peaked in popularity as a profession, and it was not unusual for almost half the students in the entering class in one prestigious ivy league school to declare that they were premedical students. Many of these students were deeply interested in science, and medical school selection committees favored students who might be attracted to careers in medical research and who were better suited to the practice of scientific medicine than their less scientific student peers.

The student unrest of the late 1960s and early 1970s, associated with opposition to the Vietnam War, caused a brief but remarkably intense concern for the social issues of medical care on the part of many medical students, sufficient to cause some to reject highly scientific subspecialty careers in favor of work as primary care physicians. The metamorphosis was short-lived and by the mid-1970s medicine had begun to lose some of its attractiveness to white males partly because the open-ended support of medical science appeared to have ended, partly because fewer students were interested in medicine as a vehicle for social reform, partly because of the length of medical training associated with an increasing debt load, and partly because of the greater attractiveness of other careers. For a time, the size of the medical applicant pool was maintained because of the increase in the number of women applying to medical school, but that pool is also diminishing. The conscious effort by medical schools to admit minorities begun in the early 1970s has been sustained, but the size of this pool of applicants also appears to be decreasing.

Clearly, a medical career is no longer as popular as it once was and this is reflected in the decline in the number of medical school applicants as well as in the attitudes of many practicing physicians today. There are two reasons for their concern: The projected excess of physicians, brought about by the doubling of medical school size as a part of federal government policy in the 1970s means that physician income is likely to decline, and physicians will no longer be able to choose where to practice without regard for the competition. The second major reason is the emphasis of the federal government on controlling medical care costs. Specifically, physicians fear that alternative practice plans will threaten further the fee-for-service system. They fear that hospitals, in response to competitive pressure, will no longer accept a passive role as the doctor's workshop and that Medicare may apply diagnosis-related groups to physician fees as well as hospital costs. In summary, they are threatened by a loss of autonomy and declining incomes, and their fears are compounded by the fear of medical malpractice suits. No wonder the sons and daughters of physicians are no longer urged to study medicine.

Policy Implications—Past and Future

As noted earlier it is impossible to change the matrix of medicine without affecting other aspects of national life and, over the course of this century, the impact has been profound. The future must be viewed from the vantage of a medical matrix that will continue to change, and since more change is inevitable, all we can do is pose the questions that are likely to become the policy issues of the decades ahead.

The past is easier. Today, government, private foundations, citizen groups, and commercial interests are all declaring an interest in the elderly, for we are rapidly becoming a society in which the demography of the nation is skewed toward the old rather than the young. That change can at least in part be attributed to medical science. There are many reasons for smaller families, one of which is the expectation that children will survive. Certainly this is a realistic expectation today thanks to the control of infectious disease. At the other end of the spectrum, people are living longer and that includes the "old-old," people over eighty years of age. This too is, to a large degree, the result of medical advance. Consider the issues raised by a change in the demography of the nation. Living longer does not necessarily mean a healthy old age, and the care of the sick elderly is a major problem. Living alone is not easy for the frail elderly and since women live longer than men, this is largely a problem for single women who are widowed, divorced, or never married. Added to this is the issue of poverty among the aged whether due to inadequate pension support, social security payments often too small to meet basic needs, or ignorance about the availability of supplemental security income. For those in poverty but ineligible for Medicaid, medical costs can also be a problem since Medicare does not cover many medical expenses. Often the only asset an elderly person has is a house, and some organizations concerned with the welfare of the elderly are examining the possibility of "reverse mortgages" as a way of mobilizing the use of this asset.

Living longer means a longer period of support on Social Security, and since there is a diminishing ratio of young to old persons, those who remain in the work force will be obligated to pay more and more into the system in order to support those who are receiving benefits. Some question the viability of the Social Security System's using the present tax base once the baby boom generation of the 1940s and 1950s reaches the age of retirement.

It may seem fanciful to attribute the sexual revolution, in part, to advances in medical science, and certainly there were many other reasons for a liberated view of sexual conduct. Nevertheless, two medical advances facilitated its inauguration: "the pill," a relatively easy way to avoid pregnancy, and penicillin, which all but eliminated the fear of syphilis and gonorrhea. One wonders about the impact of AIDS on the prevalence of sexual promiscuity now that the disease appears to be spreading into the heterosexual community and since there is no known therapy for this fatal disease.

Advances in medicine have created ethical dilemmas not previously of concern to moral philosophers. When is a birth control method an abortifacient? When is the fetus viable? What are the ethical issues created by amniocentesis and the resulting ability to diagnose genetic defects in utero? How should society view the possibility that the sex of an unborn child can be chosen in advance of artificial insemination with appropriately selected sperm? At the other end of life's spectrum, how does one define death, when is it ethical to stop life-support systems, and who should decide? These questions are being debated by religious denominations, by philosophers, by lay groups, and even by the courts. Whatever the outcomes, it is certain that patients and the families of patients will be actively involved in making decisions in concert with physicians.

An interesting dilemma has been caused by carefully performed epidemiological studies on the direct relationship between cigarettes and cancer of the lung, as well as smoking as a risk factor for cardiovascular disease and premature birth. The risks associated with cigarettes are such that if tobacco were under the purview of the federal Food and Drug Administration it would have been banned years ago. But it is not and for very good reason. Tobacco is an important crop in many states and, not only is it legal to grow tobacco, the crop is actually subsidized by the federal government. Gradually, however, there is a move to restrict the use of cigarettes, witness the recent actions to eliminate smoking by the armed forces except in certain designated areas and the increasing number of public and private buildings in which smoking is banned.

Before we consider the future let us consider some of the changes presently going on in the matrix of medicine and some questions about the direction of future change.

All hospitals, teaching and nonteaching, profit and not-for-profit are in a period of transition, and the outcome is unclear. Some will undoubtedly become parts of integrated systems of care as the Kaiser Permanente hospitals are at present, but this is unlikely for the majority. Nevertheless, hospitals will try to control as much of the delivery system as possible and will compete with physician groups for control of ambulatory surgery, and emergency and diagnostic services. They also will learn that they do not do well managing businesses unrelated to medicine. There is likely to be further attrition of hospitals, particularly small rural hospitals, and those that survive will either be highly specialized or have the capacity to provide a wide range of services. More and more hospitals will be controlled by management rather than by physician staffs.

Despite the gloomy forecasts made by many practicing physicians, the profession will continue to do well economically even if it loses some of its autonomy. The fee-for-service system is unlikely to disappear, but it will almost certainly share a larger part of the medical market with prepaid plans than is true at present. This means that more and more physicians will be salaried, at least in part.

Even though medicine remains a reasonably remunerative profession, it is probable that there will be a continuing decline in the number of qualified applicants. Those individuals who in the past were attracted to medical practice because it provided personal autonomy may well consider other careers, and the profession may become more attractive to those willing to work for large organizations and wishing to have regular hours. It is quite possible that the ratio of men to women will approach 50/50 by the start of the twenty-first century, and women who wish to combine careers in medicine with raising families are likely to find salaried positions compatible with their needs. Unless steps are taken to moderate the rising costs of a medical education, minorities and underprivileged members of the white majority will find medicine an unrealistic option as a career choice. Consequently, the profession will be drawn principally from the white middle class.

Some reform of the structure of medical education will have to be undertaken to obviate glaring redundancies in the educational process, but it is unclear what will happen to the interface between college and the first two years of medical school or between the clinical years of medical school and residency training. What the appropriate teaching environment will be also remains unresolved, although most would agree that the intensive care teaching hospital is no longer a suitable place for most clinical instruction as it is at present.

Finally, there is likely to be some redistribution of manpower among the specialties, not because of government regulation or planning on the part of the educational establishment but through the forces of the marketplace. A structured medical care system requires a greater proportion of primary care physicians than specialists, and young physicians will soon learn that more jobs are available for internists and pediatricians than for cardiac surgeons.

The question of whether medical care is a right or a privilege remains unanswered. However, some answer will have to be found to the problem of financing medical care for 35 million uninsured Americans in a competitive marketplace. The ultimate solution will probably be some form of national health insurance paid for both privately and publicly. Preoccupation with cost control will no doubt continue, and this will inevitably lead to better measures of the quality of care, greater standardization of procedures and protocols for medical practice, and greater attention to the assessment of new technologies before they are accepted in medical practice.

As medicine grows in complexity and is capable of doing more and more to alleviate the consequences of disease, to anticipate and prevent disease, and even to cure, there will be further problems of ethics and equity. Who should receive the next cardiac, liver, or kidney transplant? How does society determine the allocation of scarce resources? What are the ethics of removing organs for transplantation before the heart has stopped beating and the donor is clearly alive—an issue raised recently in the *London Times?* What guidelines need to be in place for genetic engineering that has the potential of correcting major genetic defects and who receives the benefits? These and other questions will continue to engage philosophers, religious leaders, physicians, and the general public.

The Magic of Science, Denial of Risk, and the Medicalization of Social Problems

The remarkable success of medical science has conferred on it a magical quality that is seductive for those who practice the art, but that is dangerous as well, for the expectations of patients are often too high and the denial of risk too great. There are many reasons for the malpractice crisis, but one that should not be overlooked is the denial of risk and the failure of physicians to warn adequately their patients of the risk—often considerable—of any treatment.

Medicine is not only scientific and even effective, but it is also respectable. Even the association of AIDS with homosexuality and drug addiction does not inhibit public discussion. Such openness is to be applauded, but it does not justify making almost every social problem a medical one. Teenage pregnancy is a problem and clearly sex education, instruction in the use of contraceptives, and advice about prenatal care are all important, but that does not make teenage pregnancy a medical problem. Teenage pregnancy is primarily a social problem, but a social problem is more difficult to analyze, to talk about, and to do something about so that it becomes easier to make it a medical problem.

By the time the use of hard drugs has produced addiction, a medical problem exists, but drug use is not primarily a medical problem anymore than it is a supply problem. It too is a social problem, a substantial one, and one we know very little about. It is not inherently bad to medicalize social problems, but if the medical approach diverts attention and resources away from an analysis of social issues, it postpones definitive action about these issues. Violence, crime, poverty, and homelessness are all societal problems, and while each may have some medical component, medical science will not solve any one of them.

It is impossible in this brief essay to adequately assess the changes brought about by advances in medical science. Nevertheless, the effort will have been worthwhile if the reader appreciates how medical advance inevitably changes the entire matrix of medicine and how this in turn affects many other aspects of national life. The theme is timely because we appear to have entered a period of substantial change in that medical matrix, perhaps the most dramatic since the early part of the century.

3

Allocating Health Care Resources: How Can We Ensure Access to Essential Care?

Albert L. Siu and Robert H. Brook

Public debate over the cost and quality of, and access to health care in the United States has increased in volume and intensity over the last several years as society grapples with the question of how to allocate limited health resources. Rising health costs in the past two decades have ushered in policies to contain costs. These policies have featured increasing regulation, shifting the financial burden to patients, and efforts to increase competition among health care providers. All the while, proponents and opponents have debated whether the health bill can be effectively trimmed without sacrificing quality of or access to care. Some analysts claim that current policies drive some doctors and hospitals to cut corners in the provision of care to patients; other analysts assert that we will soon have to explicitly ration access to potentially beneficial services.[1]

Meanwhile, there is evidence that resources are being wasted on useless health care while funds available for needed services are insufficient. According to a report from the Institute of Medicine, billions of dollars are spent annually on useless or unproven medical services. Concomitantly, funds are not available for the care of poor patients as evidenced by California's termination of Medicaid benefits for the medically indigent in 1982. Society also questions whether it can afford costly new technological advances in medicine, since many opponents believe that dollars could be better spent on improving access to more basic health services. Each of these controversies revolves around one question: Can our society develop ways to distribute health resources so that patients are relieved of the financial burden of high medical bills while providing access to essential or beneficial health care?

Allocating Health Care Resources

Whether explicitly or implicitly every society treats health care as a scarce or limited resource and has developed means for its allocation.

This occurs even in a wealthy society such as ours. As Fuchs has indicated, variations in surgery rates by demographic subgroups or by geographic region demonstrate the workings of a rationing mechanism.[2] Similarly—although there is no explicit policy—the type of medical care provided to our presidents is not available to all. Abundant examples of rationing are available. Insurance policies limit the services and the quantity of services they cover. Medicare purposely excludes long-term care and skilled nursing unrelated to an acute episode of illness. We have always allocated or rationed health resources in this manner, but these decisions are now becoming identifiable in terms of who makes such decisions, how they are implemented, and who is affected. Thus, the mechanisms developed to allocate health resources are coming under augmented scrutiny and criticism.

Further understanding of this controversy is found in a treatise by Calabresi and Bobbitt on how societies allot scarce resources. In their book, *Tragic Choices,* the authors maintain that societies make first-order determinations of how much will be produced and second-order determinations of who shall get what is produced.[3] The choices made by society in distributing these resources reflect prevailing norms and values. At times, choices that do not conflict with these values are possible. When this fails, however, societies are confronted with "tragic choices" and an assortment of responses to "evade, confront, or remake the tragic choice."

Using the case of renal hemodialysis as an example, U.S. policy initially avoided making a first-order determination that would place a limit on the number of hemodialysis cases to be treated. Such a determination would have conflicted with the values of this wealthiest of nations. Thus, second-order determinations were made based on "therapeutic and other efficiency considerations," and hemodialysis was allocated on the basis of whom it was "likeliest" to benefit. As long as hemodialysis was available to all who would benefit, a first-order determination could be directly avoided. However, the inability to apply second-order principles led to the failure of this strategy and to an eventual redefinition of the first-order determination so that hemodialysis was available to "all" who would benefit.

Today's debate on the cost and quality of health care parallels the history of renal hemodialysis policy. Befitting a nation with tremendous wealth, we have so far avoided making a first-order determination about how much to spend on health care. Indeed, the United States has the world's highest per capita spending on health ($1,721 in 1985) and since 1960 the percentage of gross national product devoted to health has more than doubled to 11 percent.

Consequently, allocation of health resources has been made by a series of second-order determinations. To spread the financial risk of increasingly high medical bills, indemnity and service benefit voluntary health insurance became available earlier this century and gained widespread acceptance after World War II. Although these packages were available to individual subscribers, most enrollees were employees and other low-risk groups. Confronted with the number of poor and older persons unable to obtain private insurance, the United States enacted the Medicaid and Medicare programs in 1964. For the remaining uninsured who could not afford major medical expenses, charity care (which shifted the costs to paying patients) was provided by the nation's hospitals. Through a patchwork of this type, society attempted to allocate health resources within a governing principle of equal access to all.

Within the last decade, however, the failings of this mechanism have been laid bare. Although health costs had reached staggering levels, an estimated 14 million adults remain uninsured and 4 million families claim that they do not have access to the health system when they need it.[4] To control rising costs, further second-order steps— such as prospective payment and capitation—were taken to make the health care marketplace more competitive.

Although the ultimate result of these policies is still unknown, society's uneasiness with this method of allocation has intensified. Medicare patients and their families believe that they are denied hospitalization or are prematurely discharged;[5] indigent patients are increasingly transferred from private to overburdened public hospitals;[6] and fee-for-service physicians are accusing physicians in capitated systems with rationing beneficial services for personal financial gain. All these issues conflict with our basic values and we are left with unresolved "tragic choices" on how to allocate the health dollar.

To resolve this dilemma, several options exist. One choice is to redefine the first-order determination so that all health services are universally available regardless of whether they are beneficial. Such a policy would appear unreasonable since resources would be spent on some services that have no benefit; the prohibitive cost of this option would also make it undesirable. Alternatively, more socially acceptable mechanisms that restrain resource consumption while ensuring access to essential services will need to be implemented.

Essential Care

Every method of allocation must confront the question of how to define and ensure access to essential services. At the very least, essential services include all effective diagnostic and therapeutic services, that is, services that benefit the patient when provided by the typical provider. In the strictest sense, services would not be considered effective if they are shown to be efficacious *only* in controlled circumstances. In an ideal system, effective services would not be rationed, while the use of services with no or marginal benefit would be curtailed. There is ample evidence that this is not achieved under the status quo.

In several New England communities, Wennberg et al. have reported geographic variation in the rates of performance of many surgical procedures. Comparing surgery rates in neighboring hospital service areas in New England states, they found a severalfold variation in the rate of performance of many surgical procedures, the greatest variation occurring when there were controversial or uncertain indications for a given procedure. Thus, the rate of tonsillectomy (a procedure with controversial indications) varied sixfold among the areas studied while the rate of inguinal hernia repair (a procedure with more accepted indications) varied little.[7] These variations in surgery rates did not appear to be related to differences in sociodemographic or health status.[8]

For the Medicare population, similar patterns of geographic variation in surgery rates have been demonstrated in a study of thirteen large regions of the United States (each with an average Medicare population of 340,000). For example, the rate of coronary artery bypass surgery varies from a low of 7 per 10,000 in one region to a high of 23 per 10,000 in another region.[9] Alternative treatments for the same condition demonstrated a similar pattern indicating that the variations were not due to the substitution of different therapies for the same condition. These studies suggest that the current delivery mechanism allows the performance of many services with little or unclear benefit.

More direct evidence of inappropriate medical care is available from other studies. A quarter century ago, a study of the health care received by members of a New York City union asked a panel of expert clinicians to review the medical records of those patients who had been hospitalized. The physicians found that one-fifth of the hospitalizations were unnecessary.[10] More recently, a study of the care received by Medicare and Medicaid patients in four regions of the United States found that one in five hospitalizations was inappropriate.[11]

In the Rand Health Insurance Experiment, a study which randomly assigned families in six sites across the United States to insurance plans with different levels of cost sharing, the medical records of all adults who had been hospitalized (excluding pregnancy) during 1975–1982 were reviewed. The physicians, reviewing 1,132 hospital records, found that one in five adult non-Medicare hospitalizations and one in three hospital days were inappropriate in that acute hospital services were either not provided or were unnecessary; an additional one in five hospitalizations could have been avoided through the substitution of ambulatory surgical services.[12] For the most part, this study considered only the appropriateness of the hospital setting and whether acute hospital services were provided. If acute hospital services were provided, we did not label as inappropriate hospitalizations where the medical indications for performing a given procedure were uncertain or not present. Thus, a hysterectomy could be considered appropriate if surgery was performed in a timely manner even though the medical indications for the procedure were controversial.

If we also appraise the efficacy of a procedure, many more hospitalizations would be considered inappropriate. Consider carotid endarterectomy, a procedure performed six times more frequently today than a decade ago. A recent study asked a panel of experts to rate the appropriateness of 864 potential clinical indications for this procedure. Based on the panel ratings, only 55 percent of the carotid endarterectomies performed in five Veterans Administration teaching hospitals were clearly appropriate (13 percent were inappropriate and one-third were performed for equivocal indications). If one also took into consideration the provider's rate of perioperative complications and the patient's age, functional status, and life expectancy only 23 percent of the surgeries would have been considered appropriate.[13] In another study of coronary angiography and coronary artery bypass surgery performed in community hospitals, preliminary results indicate that about one-half of these procedures are performed for clearly appropriate medical indications (a quarter are equivocal and the remainder are inappropriate).[14] These studies indicate that current allocating mechanisms fail to filter out many questionable surgical procedures.

At the same time, some third-party payers have been reluctant to cover beneficial services. Fearing uncontrolled utilization, third parties have been unwilling to cover preventive services and selected other services that are clearly beneficial to health. Standard Medicare benefits, for example, do not cover visual and hearing aids even though visual disorders are prevalent in 14 percent and hearing disorders in 28 percent of older persons. Similarly, coverage for certain rehabilitative services in the Medicare program sometimes cannot be obtained for frail patients with chronic multifactorial disabilities because they do not have any of several specific diagnoses that qualify for such services.

Analogously, third-party payers have been hesitant to cover sound experimental "big-ticket" treatments. Although these technologies might have formidable pricetags, their cost-effectiveness might compare quite favorably with that of other less-expensive services. Consider the case of heart transplants. Casscells has reported that this procedure costs approximately $125,000 to perform or $23,000 to $33,700 per added year of life; this compares with $10,000 per year for coronary-artery bypass surgery, $32,000 per year for hemodialysis, and $30,000 per year for screening and treatment of hypertension.[15] However, third-party payers, prepaid plans, and the government were concerned about the implications of covering heart transplants; in fact, many plans did not cover the procedure for many years. The same case could be made for liver and bone marrow transplants. Coverage was not available for many of these procedures, even though they were scientifically sound and were being developed under strict study protocols.

Thus, what we mean by essential services is really twofold. One is medical services of proven efficacy. The ideal system would reduce the use of inappropriate services with little or no efficacy and would guarantee access to efficacious services. Our notion of essential care must also recognize that for many conditions efficacious treatments do not exist or existing treatments need to be improved. As such, essential care must include the timely provision of experimental services or new technologies in controlled settings where appropriateness and outcome can be rigorously evaluated.

Effectiveness of Current Mechanisms

How well do existing rationing mechanisms ensure access to essential services? Many attempts to limit health expenditures have been and are being attempted. These include deductibles and copayments, prepayments, caps or overall limits on hospital expenditures, primary care gatekeepers, incentives to direct care to preferred providers, and prospective payment based on diagnosis-related groups (DRGs). Although there is insufficient empirical evidence on how all these methods will perform, there are sufficient data to suspect that these methods alone are unlikely to ensure access to essential care.

In the last several years, cost sharing by consumers has been widely used to reduce health costs. In 1982, 67 percent of insurance plans covered hospital care at no cost to patients. By 1984, this percentage had decreased to 42 percent.[16] Although cost sharing is effective in reducing costs, results from the Rand Health Insurance Experiment indicate that it does not ensure access to effective care in that it reduces use of both essential and nonessential services. In the study discussed earlier, we found that cost sharing resulted in proportional reductions in both appropriate and inappropriate hospitalization.[17] With respect to ambulatory visits, cost sharing generally resulted in similar reductions in visits for general medical exams, acute or chronic problems. Similarly, visits were equally reduced whether they were for conditions where medical care was or was not effective. Surprisingly, cost sharing did not negatively affect health; this suggests that the negative effects expected from reduced effective services were balanced by positive effects resulting from the reductions in noneffective services with associated iatrogenesis.[18] Perhaps these results are not surprising since cost sharing places much of the burden of allocating on patients who may not be informed about what conditions can or cannot be effectively treated.

Prepaid group practice, on the other hand, places most allocating decisions on health care providers who sometimes have a financial incentive to limit utilization. Whether these organizations are able to selectively reduce inappropriate care, however, remains inconclusive. In his synthesis of the literature, Luft found that health maintenance organizations (HMOs) reduced utilization "across the board."[19] He found that compared to their fee-for-service counterparts HMOs achieved equal reductions in surgical and nonsurgical admissions, and that they did not disproportionately reduce admissions for certain categories of diagnoses that might be considered discretionary. For example, he found that prepaid plans reduced hysterectomies (which might be considered a more discretionary procedure) and other admissions to a similar extent. In another study comparing physicians in fee-for-service and prepaid practices, LoGerfo et al. found that prepayment reduced both necessary and unnecessary surgical procedures.[20] Other studies, however, have shown that HMOs are able to select areas for reductions. For example, the care of patients with colorectal cancer and rheumatoid arthritis is relatively similar in prepaid and fee-for-service settings.[21] As with cost sharing, prepayment effectively reduces health costs; however, it remains unclear whether reductions in utilization are achieved selectively. Furthermore, there is no reason to believe that prepaid systems per se will be able to improve responses to how new costly technologies are to be introduced.

To reduce unnecessary surgery, second opinions have been advocated for elective procedures. However, whether such programs reduce necessary (as well as unnecessary) surgery is not known. The programs reduce the rates of surgery beyond what one would attribute directly to second opinions, that is, the mere existence of such programs reduces the number of surgeries proposed;[22] whether fewer necessary procedures are proposed is not known. Furthermore, when the second opinion fails to confirm the need for surgery and third opinions are sought, the second opinion is reversed 70 percent of the time.[23] This would indicate that some of the second opinions would have excluded necessary surgery and/or that this mechanism fails to reduce surgery in questionable instances.

Lacking empirical data, we can only speculate about the consequences of other policy options. To control costs in the state's Medi-Cal (Medicaid) program, California terminated Medi-Cal coverage in 1982 for indigent adults not eligible for federal assistance programs; the medical care for these individuals was transferred to the counties' public hospital system. A study of the individuals affected at one medical center found that termination from Medi-Cal had adversely affected access to the health care system, patient satisfaction, health status, and control of hypertension. Whereas 3 percent of individuals had diastolic blood pressures exceeding 100 mm Hg while on Medi-Cal, six months after termination 31 percent had diastolic pressures exceeding this level.[24] We can reasonably assume that these negative health consequences were at least partly the result of lost access to effective services. Indeed, although four out of five of these individuals believed that they could obtain medical care whenever it was needed under Medicaid, only two of five felt they could six months after Medicaid termination.

It is too early to assess the effects of prospective payment and other policies such as preferred provider groups. If preferred providers were chosen on the basis of their clinical expertise, one could argue that the allocation of services would improve—that is effective services would be assured and unnecessary care would be curtailed by these preferred providers. To the best of our knowledge, however, providers will be "preferred" not on the basis of clinical expertise but on the cost of their style of practice.

Prospective payment appears to have been successful in reducing hospital use, and peer review organizations are attempting to monitor for and reduce inappropriate use of the hospital for nonacute purposes. However, whether they will be successful in reducing surgical procedures (or other acute hospital services) that may not be medically necessary is less clear. As with other approaches, prospective payment per se also has no provisions for ensuring the orderly acquisition and evaluation of therapies.

An Alternative Approach

Given the delivery of many inappropriate services in the face of inadequate funding for other needed services, the central challenge to any system of allocation will be to effect a better distribution of health resources and services. Existing mechanisms allocate health resources on the basis of economic or administrative constraints. As such, it is our contention that neither of the existing mechanisms—namely cost sharing and prepayment—alone is sufficient to resolve the "tragic choice" confronting U.S. society. To do so, we believe that clinical guidelines need to be incorporated into a mechanism to allocate health services to accomplish the following objectives:

- Protect individuals from the financial burden of large medical bills.
- Limit costs to a level acceptable to society.

- Provide access for all to efficacious and effective medical care.
- When therapy of sufficient efficacy does not exist, provide access to experimental care and the scientific evaluation of such care.
- Advance medical knowledge on the efficacy of alternative medical services by evaluating existing and new technologies.
- Minimize inappropriate use of medical services.

The first four objectives have been discussed above. The last two objectives are critical to the success of the overall approach. An allocating mechanism that is based on clinical guidelines and the efficacy of services cannot succeed without more information on the circumstances in which specific services are effective. Similarly, if broader access to services is to be made available, cost savings must be realized through selective reductions in the use of inappropriate services. In addition to freeing resources for services with greater utility, reduction of inappropriate care would reduce negative iatrogenic outcomes.

How might a prototypical package be structured? Coverage of specific services or procedures could be limited to specific clinical indications determined by professional consensus. For many procedures—selected on the basis of clinical and cost considerations—coverage would be limited to clinical indications where the benefit of performing the procedure exceeded the negative consequences (e.g., mortality and morbidity) associated with the procedure. For example, coverage for coronary artery bypass surgery or carotid endarterectomy might be limited to patients with specific clinical presentations and angiographic findings. These indications would include circumstances in which the services had been shown to be efficacious and, if insufficient data existed, to those circumstances in which efficacy could be expected based on professional consensus. Thus, carotid endarterectomy might not be covered for certain patients. Obtaining such consensus on the indications for a variety of surgical procedures is feasible.[25] Such a process would eliminate inappropriate surgery and would identify surgery for equivocal indications. For lack of adequate information on effectiveness, some of the equivocal procedures might be covered. In some cases, the outcome (e.g., mortality or repeat surgery) of patients treated for equivocal indications might be followed. At any rate, knowing the frequency of equivocal indications would permit an enlightened dialogue in approaching this issue.

Many services will not warrant the specification of indications since they are either inexpensive, clearly efficacious, or unlikely to be abused. Examples of such services might include the casting of an extremity fracture, the incision and drainage of abscesses, and surgery for acute abdominal conditions. Some procedures demonstrated to be useless would not be covered under any circumstance. An example of such a procedure would include extracranial-intracranial artery bypass, surgery that has been recently shown to have no efficacy in the treatment of cerebrovascular disease.[26]

For many medical conditions and specific clinical circumstances, rigorous scientific information about the efficacy of care is not known. For some of these circumstances, randomized (or nonrandomized) evaluation of the efficacy of existing or new therapies may be appropriate. If warranted by cost or other clinical issues, selected services might be covered only if performed under controlled circumstances that would permit follow-up and evaluation of outcome. With such a mechanism, improved information would be available to update consensus judgments on the clinical indications for given procedures. Consensus on clinical indications would be facilitated by more information on efficacy. Similarly, new technologies accompanied by careful monitoring of efficacy could be introduced.

Certainly many procedures will continue to be performed without studies documenting their efficacy. In this sense, the above scenario is not unlike the status quo. Unique clinical circumstances at times will require departure from the above framework; thus, a process for judicious appeal of disputes over coverage will be required. Of course, an innovation of this type is a huge undertaking. However, the process could be phased in over years and could complement either prospective payment initiatives, fee-for-service arrangements, or prepaid reimbursement.

In the belief that increasing rules and regulations of this genre would work "clumsily," Thurow has advocated that the medical profession deal with health spending issues by developing new norms of behavior that recognize the need to balance both the costs and benefits of health services.[27] This, in effect, is similar to what we propose with the exception that the allocating criteria would be internalized by physicians and no explicit criteria would exist. In view of the paucity of data on the costs and benefits of most medical treatments, we argue that Thurow's approach would have little chance of success. Rather, the approach we advocate would establish both a formal process for linking benefits with efficacy and a system for obtaining greater information on efficacy.

Clearly, this approach focuses heavily on the so-called "big-ticket" items—hospitalizations and major surgical procedures. It would be inappropriate for controlling unnecessary utilization and ensuring appropriate utilization for many other services such as laboratory tests, radiologic procedures, and drug treatments. Many of these procedures (e.g., gastrointestinal contrast studies and treadmill tests) and treatments (e.g., chronic treatment of hypertension and diabetes) have important implications for cost and quality; yet, the approach advocated above would probably be excessively bureaucratic to apply to these frequently performed "small-ticket" items. To ensure the appropriate mix of these services, a voluntary program featuring a combination of medical record audit with incentives for good performance might be implemented by major medical societies or licensing boards. Guidelines for the treatment of common clinical conditions could be developed, a sample of a provider's medical records could be audited periodically, and rewards (e.g., advancement in a medical society or exemption from a recertification exam) could be given for good performance.

Many people might say that this amounts to a "cookbook" approach to medicine. We would argue, however, that such an approach is already used widely and accepted in medicine. One need look only at successive editions of the *Washington University Manual on Medical Therapeutics*, the "pocket Bible" of medical interns and residents, currently in its 25th edition, to affirm this fact;[28] in it one finds explicit guidelines on the management of a variety of disorders ranging from diabetic ketoacidosis to gonococcal urethritis. Medicine has become sufficiently vast and complicated, technology changes sufficiently fast, and the magnitude of public resources expended sufficiently large, to warrant the explication of such guidelines and the implementation of a system of voluntary audits and incentives. Respecting coverage of heart transplants, the federal government has specified clinical indications for coverage in a process similar to that which we propose.

The development of a monitoring system would appear particularly necessary in view of a current trend favoring potential underutilization of beneficial services. The environment for such underutilization is created by the incentives inherent in prepayment and in DRG-based prospective payment. Thus, an auditing system such as outlined above could serve as a check against both overutilization and underutilization.

To ensure against underutilization, however, a voluntary plan may need to be complemented by a monitoring system with limited mandatory audits triggered by the occurrence of certain adverse or sentinel events. One could envision a system to monitor for sentinel health events—defined as potentially preventable outcomes the occurrence of which should lead to an investigation of the care rendered. A listing of such sentinel events (e.g., death from diabetic ketoacidosis or Hodgkin's Disease) was prepared by Rutstein et al. several years ago and could be updated and modified for this purpose.[29] The occurrence of a sentinel event or events above a certain threshold rate might trigger an audit of the involved hospitals or physicians.

Will the proposal we advance avert the impending rationing of beneficial services described by other commentators? Technological advance annually produces new and expensive procedures. Meanwhile, the aging of the U.S. population is expected to increase significantly health service utilization in the coming decades. Nonetheless, we believe that rationing of beneficial services is not inevitable if methods to reduce nonessential care selectively could be developed. Be that as it may, we acknowledge that we may be wrong and that the succession of technologic and geriatric imperatives may raise health costs to a level exceeding that which society is willing to pay; in that case, rationing of beneficial services may be inevitable as others have suggested. If this circumstance arises, however, we contend that we will still need to develop methods to reduce inappropriate or marginally effective services. It would be desirable to reduce such services before rationing essential care.

Our proposal may appear excessive and revolutionary to some; however, the evidence suggests that U.S. society is confronting a *tragic choice* respecting its spending on health. Our current system offends the values of some, and our spending priorities are questioned. There are those who decry the increasing presence of the profit motive in medical practice;[30] others question whether contemporary physicians can continue to act in the best interests of their patients.[31] And while our per capita health expenditure is the highest among large industrialized nations, we are confronted with the potential rationing of beneficial treatments while providing many treatments of dubious or unknown value. As we have argued here, the tried and proven mechanisms for rationing health care are unlikely to yield acceptable solutions. Thus, a dialogue is needed on innovative approaches to contain costs while ensuring access to essential services. This paper represents our attempt to forge a clinical response to this question.

Notes

1. H. J. Aaron and W. B. Schwartz, *The Painful Prescription: Rationing Hospital Care* (Washington, D.C.: Brookings Institution, 1984); and R. W. Evans, "Health Care Technology and the Inevitability of Resource Allocation and Rationing Decisions," *Journal of the American Medical Association* 249 (1983):2047–2053, 2208–2219.

2. V. R. Fuchs, "The 'Rationing' of Medical Care," *New England Journal of Medicine* 311 (1984):1572–1573.

3. G. Calabresi and P. Bobbitt, *Tragic Choices* (New York: W.W. Norton and Co., 1978).

4. Robert Wood Johnson Foundation, *Special Report: Updated Report on Access to Health Care for the American People* (Princeton: Robert Wood Johnson Foundation, 1983).

5. U.S. Senate, Special Committee on Aging, *Impact of Medicare's Prospective*

Payment System on the Quality of Care Received by Medicare Beneficiaries, Staff Report (Washington, D.C.: Special Committee on Aging, John Heinz, Chairman, October 24, 1985).

6. R. L. Schiff et al., "Transfers to a Public Hospital. A Prospective Study of 467 Patients," *New England Journal of Medicine* 314 (1986):552–556.

7. J. E. Wennberg and A. Gittlesohn, "Variations in Medical Care Among Small Areas," *Scientific American* 246 (1982):120–134.

8. J. E. Wennberg and J. F. Fowler, Jr., "A Test of Consumer Contribution to Small Area Variations in Health Care Delivery," *Journal of the Maine Medical Association* 68 (1977):275–279.

9. M. R. Chassin et al., "Variations in the Use of Medical and Surgical Services by the Medicare Population," *New England Journal of Medicine* 314 (1986):285–290.

10. M. A. Moorehead and R. Donaldson, *A Study of the Quality of Hospital Care Secured by a Sample of Teamsters' Family Members in New York City* (New York: Columbia University, School of Public Health and Administrative Medicine, 1964).

11. J. D. Restuccia et al., "The Appropriateness of Hospital Use," *Health Affairs* 3 (1984):130–138.

12. A. L. Siu et al., "Inappropriate Use of Hospitals in a Randomized Trial of Health Insurance Plans," *New England Journal of Medicine* 315 (1986):1259–1266.

13. N. J. Merrick et al., "Use of Carotid Endarterectomy in Five California Veteran Administration Medical Centers," *Journal of the American Medical Association* 256 (1986):2531–2535; and N. J. Merrick et al., "Derivation of Clinical Indications for Carotid Endarterectomy by an Expert Panel," *American Journal of Public Health* 77 (1987) 187–190.

14. C. M. Winslow et al., "The Appropriateness of Use of Coronary Angiography and Coronary Artery Bypass Surgery," *Clinical Research* 34 (1986):635A.

15. W. Casscells, "Heart Transplantation," *New England Journal of Medicine* 315 (1986):1365–1368.

16. J. Goldsmith, "Death of a Paradigm: The Challenge of Competition," *Health Affairs* 3 (1984):5–19.

17. Siu et al., "Inappropriate Use of Hospitals."

18. K. N. Lohr et al., "Use of Medical Care in the Rand Health Insurance Experiment: Diagnosis and Service Specific Analyses in a Randomized Controlled Trial," *Medical Care* 24 (1986):S1–S87.

19. H. S. Luft, "How Do Health Maintenance Organizations Achieve Their Savings?" *New England Journal of Medicine* 298 (1978):1336–1343.

20. J. P. LoGerfo et al., "Rates of Surgical Care in Prepaid Group Practices and the Independent Setting: What are the Reasons for the Differences?"*Medical Care* 17 (1979):1–7.

21. E. H. Yelin, M. A. Shearn, and W. V. Epstein, "Health Outcomes for a Chronic Disease in Prepaid Group Practice and Fee-for-Service Settings," *Medical Care* 24 (1986):236–246; and A. M. Francis, L. Pollisar, A. B. Lorenz, "Care of Patients with Colorectal Cancer: A Comparison of a Health Maintenance Organization and Fee-for-Service Practices," *Medical Care* 22 (1984):418–429.

22. S. G. Martin et al., "Impact of a Mandatory Second-Opinion Program on Medicaid Surgery Rates," *Medical Care* 20 (1982):21–45.

23. P. M. Gertman et al., "Second Opinions for Elective Surgery," *New England Journal of Medicine* 302 (1980):1169–1174.

24. N. Lurie et al., "Termination from Medi-Cal—Does It Affect Health?" *New England Journal of Medicine* 311 (1984):480–484.

25. R. E. Park et al., "Physician Ratings of Appropriate Indications for Six Medical and Surgical Procedures," *American Journal of Public Health* 76 (1986):766–772.

26. F. Plum, "Extracranial-Intracranial Arterial Bypass and Cerebral Vascular Disease," *New England Journal of Medicine* 313 (1985):1221–1223; and EC/IC Bypass Study Group, "Failure of Extracranial-Intracranial Arterial Bypass to Reduce the Risk of Ischemic Stroke," *New England Journal of Medicine* 313 (1985):1191–1200.

27. L. C. Thurow, "Learning to Say 'No'," *New England Journal of Medicine* 311 (1984):1569–1572.

28. M. J. Orland and R. J. Saltman, eds., *Manual of Medical Therapeutics, 25th Edition* (Boston: Little Brown and Co., 1986).

29. D. D. Rutstein et al., "Measuring the Quality of Medical Care," *New England Journal of Medicine* 294 (1976):582–588.

30. A. S. Relman, "The Future of Medical Practice," *Health Affairs* 2 (1983):5–19.

31. N. G. Levinsky, "The Doctor's Master," *New England Journal of Medicine* 311 (1985):1573–1575.

4

Alternative Treatments and Outcomes for Patients with Cardiovascular Diseases

J.G.G. Ledingham

Choices among medical treatments when the results of such treatment are well known and beyond doubt are few, for instance, penicillin for pneumococcal disease or standard drugs for active tuberculosis. It is quite another matter when outcome is uncertain. Treatments then have to be compared by controlled clinical trials. Although such trials are valuable, the results are strictly applicable only to the population treated (which is often atypical) under the precise circumstances of the trial.[1] Many clinical trials do not include sufficient numbers of patients for the study to adequately detect small advantages or disadvantages in treatment. Under these circumstances, apparently conflicting data are published, allowing clinicians freedom to prescribe what they think best for particular patients in particular circumstances. Choice of treatment then is influenced by the availability of technological resources, the personal expertise of the physician, medical fashion and cultural influences, the expectations of the patient, and increasingly, concerns for "quality of life." Sadly, the method of remuneration of the doctor has also been shown to be a determinant of choice of treatment.

Hypertension

Malignant Phase

The syndrome of malignant hypertension is one of the few cardiovascular disorders in which treatment is fairly uniform and outcome known. Before the development of effective antihypertensive drugs in the early 1950s, the risk to the hypertensive population of developing the malignant phase was around 7 percent. At that time the one-year mortality from the condition was about 90 percent; and since two-thirds of the patients who died were in uremia, the quality of life was also considerably impaired. Within a few years after the introduction of ganglion-blocking drugs, the proportion of hypertensives who developed the malignant phase had decreased to 1 percent, and now it is a disappearing disease in countries with developed medical services, although still a problem in other parts of the world. Recent estimates suggest a five-year survival rate for at least 85 percent of these increasingly rare victims.[2] Against such a background, there is an urgent need for prompt administration of antihypertensive drugs in such cases. Treatment is remarkably uniform among physicians and throughout the United States, Sweden, and Great Britain, and outcome is also remarkably uniform.

Severe Hypertension

In the category of hypertension classed as "severe" but short of the malignant phase (defined as diastolic pressures always in excess of 115 mmHg) there is again little heterogeneity in medical practice despite the criticisms which have been leveled at the clinical trials on which such treatment is based. Apart from a proper concern that recorded pressures be an accurate reflection of the subjects' blood pressure at home or at work and not an alarm reaction, few would doubt the need to prescribe antihypertensive drugs. The aim of such treatment is to prevent stroke, heart failure, and myocardial infarction. Evidence suggests that this therapy has been successful in the first two diseases. Between 1950 and 1974 death from stroke fell by 32 percent in the United States and by 15-20 percent in England and Wales. The rate has been declining also in Australia and in New Zealand but not in Eastern Europe (Bulgaria, Czechoslovakia, Rumania, Poland, Hungary). While the decline had begun before the advent of useful antihypertensive measures, in both the United States and New Zealand the decrease in the rate of death from stroke accelerated in the 1970s when more attention was given to detection and treatment of raised arterial pressure.

The evidence that morbidity or mortality from coronary artery disease among severe hypertensives has been significantly reduced by antihypertensive treatment is at best debatable despite the claims of the Hypertension Detection and Follow-Up Program (HDFP) study.[3] In two recent reports from hypertension clinics in the United Kingdom, the risk of death despite treatment was two to five times that expected for appropriate age and sex.[4] Ischemic heart disease was responsible for one-third of the deaths and stroke for one-fifth. The possibility that thiazide diuretics, commonly prescribed at too high a dose in hypertensives, might by their metabolic ill effects tend to provoke coronary artery disease has been quite carefully considered. No such effect can be distinguished, and the current perception is that preventing smoking may be more efficacious in protecting against myocardial infarction than better control of arterial pressure or the selection of antihypertensive drugs with supposedly "cardioprotective" effects.

Lesser degrees of hypertension pose greater problems in assessing the relationship between treatment and outcome. This is an area in which divergent views are held and in which consensus has not yet been achieved.[5]

Mild Hypertension

Between 1975 and 1985, particularly in the United States, physicians tended to use drugs to lower arterial pressure among the huge number (20-25 million in the United States) whose untreated diastolic blood pressures lay between 90 and 100 mmHg. The argument rested at least to some degree on extrapolation from data confirming the beneficial effects of treatment of higher pressures and on the suggestion from epidemiologists that a small reduction of blood pressure in the large number of people with "mild" hypertension might prevent more deaths from stroke and myocardial infarction than would more vigorous treatment of the smaller number of people with higher pressures. This calculation of course makes the unwarranted assumption that the risk associated with the untreated pressure can be reduced to that associated with the posttreatment pressure. In fact there is no evidence that such is the case; indeed, untreated subjects with mild hypertension have a better prognosis than those who have only achieved that pressure by drug therapy.

The data available before publication of the Medical Research Council (MRC) trial of treatment in mild hypertension did not help to reconcile opposing views about whether patients with arterial pressures in excess of 140/90 really benefited from treatment.[6] The doubters would emphasize the results of the Australian National Blood Pressure Study and the Oslo Study.[7] The Australian study reported on approximately 3,500 patients aged between thirty-five and sixty-five with diastolic pressures of 95-109 mmHg. Although treatment with drugs favorably influenced the incidence of fatal and nonfatal stroke, there was little difference between treatment and placebo groups with respect to clinical manifestations of coronary disease (Table 4.1), which is the greatest hazard of mild hypertension.

The Oslo study included 785 men with systolic pressures of 150-180 and diastolics of 90-110 mmHg. Active treatment reduced the incidence of stroke, heart failure, and dissecting aneurysm; seven strokes occurred among patients who received placebos and none in the group who received drug therapy. Treatment had no effect on the incidence of coronary disease despite an average difference of 17/10 mmHg in pres-

TABLE 4.1
Data from the Australian National Blood Pressure Study

	Drug Treatment	Placebo
Deaths from coronary artery disease	5	11
Nonfatal myocardial infarctions	28	22
Total	33	33

Source: Australian National Blood Pressure Study.

sures between those who received treatment and those given placebos. Indeed, the number of deaths from coronary disease was greater in the treatment group (six) than in the control group (two).

In the Hypertension Detection and Follow-Up Program (HDFP), some 8,000 patients with initial diastolic pressures between 90 and 105 were studied by comparing intensive and expert overall medical care (stepped-care) with routine community care (referred care). In this population, mortality from cardiovascular disorders after five years was 26 percent lower in the intensively treated than in the referred-care group. According to death certificate analysis, the incidence of myocardial infarction was 45 percent less in the intensively treated group. This figure may exaggerate the true difference since a number of deaths were reported under the imprecise title of "other ischemic heart disease;" in this category 10 percent more deaths occurred in the intensively treated group. Some researchers have concluded that this evidence is enough to make mandatory the treatment of all subjects with arterial pressures exceeding 140/90 mmHg. Opponents point out the unusual nature of HDFP, a trial which has not been accepted in any large degree outside the United States. For instance, this was not a trial of specific drug treatment versus no treatment for those at risk. The stepped-care group received free transport to clinics and was carefully advised about the effects of smoking, diet, and weight. What contribution derived from excellent and free care over and above the effects of antihypertensive drugs is uncertain. Many would consider that stopping smoking was likely to have had a more beneficial effect than antihypertensive treatment. The mortality rates in HDFP in general were high; for instance, the rates of death from all causes for those with diastolic pressures of 90-95 mmHg were 7 per 1,000 patient years in the stepped-care group and 10.6 per 1,000 in the referred-care group. These figures are much higher than for comparable groups in the Australian trial. How many of the referred-care patients developed more severe hypertension without detection or treatment? Analogy from other trials in which placebo-treated patients were given treatment if pressures rose beyond an acceptable level suggests that some 2 percent might have been at risk in the referred-care group. These reservations about HDFP and the findings of the Multiple Risk Factor Intervention Trial (MRFIT) study[8] that patients with preexisting ECG abnormalities who received special intervention had a higher rate of coronary deaths than those left to "usual care," are more consistent with the previous trials and the 1985 MRC trial of mild hypertension.[9]

Much had been expected of the MRC study, a carefully conducted and costly trial which involved a single blind assessment of drug treatment versus placebo in 17,354 subjects aged thirty-five to sixty-five with initial diastolic pressures of 90-105 mmHg observed over an average of five-and-a-half years. This provided data equivalent to 85,572 patient years of observation. There was random allocation to fixed dose bendrofluazide 10 mg daily versus placebo or up to 240 mg propranolol versus placebo. Methyldopa or guanethidine were added in cases in which active drugs had not lowered diastolic pressure below the target of 90 mmHg.

Drug therapy was associated with fewer fatal strokes (18 versus 27) and with substantially fewer total strokes (60 versus 109). As in previous trials and in contrast to HDFP, there was no difference in cardiac or noncardiac deaths and among women mortality from all causes was higher in the treated group in which there were also more malignancies. An often-quoted summary of results is that drug treatment of 850 patients for one year would be expected to prevent one stroke, but would have no effect on the incidence of myocardial infarction. There are obvious reservations to that too-simple message. For instance, results were analyzed on an "intention to treat" basis, but 44 percent of the men and 37 percent of the women stopped the treatment to which they had been originally assigned. In the placebo groups 20 percent of males and 15 percent of females came to treatment because of increasingly high arterial pressures. Even so, the results of this important trial do not support the decision to treat all those with pressures over 140/90, particularly in the light of the remarkably high rate of side effects in the treated groups. The trend on both sides of the Atlantic is toward much greater selectivity among patients with borderline pressures; it is believed that treatment should be considered only for those in whom there are other risk factors or an ominous family history. Most physicians would recommend a long period of observation, exclusion of alarm reaction "pseudohypertension," and a trial of nonpharmacological approaches before introducing drug treatment. In light of the low benefit to disadvantage ratio at this level of blood pressure, there is also increasing awareness of the need to prescribe drugs which do not detract from the day-to-day sensation of good health perceived by the untreated subject. In reducing the incidence of stroke and myocardial infarction, the greater importance of preventing smoking and excess consumption of alcohol than of assaulting the borderline pressure with drugs is increasingly recognized.

Nonpharmacological Treatment of Mild Hypertension

Obesity. Obesity and hypertension are correlated in cross-sectional studies. Moreover, those who gain weight rapidly when young appear to be at a greater risk of hypertension later. The balance of data suggests that weight loss in the obese is associated with a fall in pressure, but the effect is often small. Whether lowering blood pressure by weight reduction is more or less effective in preventing cardiovascular disease remains to be seen.

Dietary salt. National advisory bodies have stated that salt restriction is a useful method of reducing the prevalence of hypertension and by implication, its complications, but there is considerable controversy about this claim and a number of questions remain.[10] For instance, does salt restriction prevent hypertension or does it only ameliorate it once it is established? If it does lower high pressures, is it effective in all, some, or in what proportion of the hypertensive population? Will the lowering of arterial pressure by dietary salt restriction reduce the incidence of stroke as does drug treatment? How far should intake be reduced to maintain optimum balance between the prevention of cardiovascular disease on the one hand and unnecessary dietary restriction on the other? Are there any harmful effects of dietary salt restriction, for instance, volume depletion in the elderly, in compulsive exercisers, and in those exposed to high temperatures? Recent data suggest that salt restriction is most effective in those with the highest pressures and least so in those with borderline values. This last finding is disappointing since it is in the borderline group that nonpharmacological approaches will be most commonly applied.

There can be no objection to moderate restriction of dietary salt, but evidence that this is predictably beneficial in prevention of coronary disease or stroke is unproven.

Alcohol. A connection between heavy drinking and hypertension is well recognized. Withdrawal from heavy drinking can markedly reduce arterial pressure and continued drinking can aggravate it. Indeed, there is an increasingly recognized association between high alcohol consumption, paroxysmal hypertension, and stroke or transient ischemic attack. There are many reasons to advocate reduction in alcohol intake but one of the least recognized is the beneficial effects on arterial pressure which may ensue.

Calcium. The evidence that low consumption of calcium in the diet is truly implicated in the etiology of hypertension or that calcium or vitamin D supplements might reduce arterial pressure is too slim. Observations in this area include increased urinary calcium, reduced plasma ionized calcium, or increased serum PTH concentration. Claims that oral calcium loading might initiate a reduction in arterial pressure need confirmation.

Exercise. There is now evidence that a program of quite simple physical training, for instance Canadian Air Force exercises, can reduce arterial pressure significantly although the long-term influence of exercise on cardiovascular morbidity and mortality cannot be accurately assessed on the basis of present data.

Vegetarian diets. Arterial pressure is lower in vegetarians than in omnivores and a strict vegetarian diet for normotensive and hypertensive individuals previously eating animal products has been shown to lower arterial pressure in at least three studies. Multiple factors are probably involved and it would be premature to suggest vegetarianism as an effective approach to the treatment of borderline hypertension.

Biofeedback and relaxation techniques. Although there are reports of relaxation techniques resulting in significant and remarkably sustained decreases in arterial pressure such studies have involved small numbers of subjects. It is even possible that pressure is lowered successfully only in "pseudohypertensives," i.e., those with a brisk alarm reaction, in whom long-term prognosis is probably benign in any case.

In relation to these various nonpharmacological approaches to the treatment of hypertension, the Hypertension Control Program (HCP) has recently reported the results of a four-year randomized controlled trial of the effects of nutritional advice on arterial pressure in patients withdrawn from drug therapy which had previously controlled pressures well.[11] In the nutritionally advised group, particular attention was paid to weight reduction and sodium and alcohol restriction. A second group simply had drugs withdrawn and a third continued on drug treatment. Some 39 percent of those exposed to nutritional advice remained normotensive at four years in contrast to 5 percent of those not so advised. These results give a further boost to a developing trend toward nonpharmacological therapy of mild hypertension.

Coronary Artery Disease

Prevention

Coronary artery disease (CAD) is the leading cause of death in the United Kingdom, responsible for one-third of all deaths among men and one-quarter among women. Some parts of Britain, e.g., Scotland, Northern Ireland, and Wales, have higher rates than others. The slight decline in death rates from coronary disease in the United Kingdom since 1979, most evident in men aged thirty-five to forty-four, is unimpressive compared to the steep fall which has been and is occuring in the United States. Rates for men have been declining also in Canada, Australia, New Zealand, Belgium, Norway, Finland, and the Netherlands. But the rates of coronary disease among men have been increasing in Sweden and in the countries of Eastern Europe. Among women rates seem to be declining everywhere (Figures 4.1 and 4.2).[12]

The rapid decline in the rate of death from CAD in the United States has been attributed to changes in life-style, particularly diet, exercise, and smoking habits. Certainly these have changed much more and much earlier than in the United Kingdom, despite the recommendations of the Committee on Medical Aspects of Food Policy (COMA) in 1974, the joint report of the Royal College of Physicians and the British Cardiac Society in 1976, and the second COMA report in 1977.[13] There was no decrease in the proportion of energy in the diet derived from fat in Britain between 1970 and 1980. It remained at around 42 percent although there was a trend toward less saturated and more polyunsaturated fat. The polyunsaturated to saturated (PS) ratio increased from 0.2 to 0.27 compared with 0.5 in the United States. Foods have not been labeled with nutritional content in the United Kingdom and medical as well as lay skepticism is widespread.[14] Aspects of the Common Market Food Policy favoring dairy farming may have contributed to the lack of change.

This is in marked contrast to the state of affairs in the United States where intake of dietary fat has dropped and linoleic acid has greatly increased. The major part of the reason is surely cultural. Alfred Yarrow has suggested that the shadow of John Stuart Mill may be responsible for the rather British view that the advice to change traditional diets is an infringement of personal liberty. In this context he quotes from Mill: ". . . That the only purpose for which power can be rightly exercised over any members of a civilised community against his will, is to prevent harm to others. His own good, either physical or moral is not a sufficient warrant."[15]

British skepticism persists despite the country's "top of the table" position in world rankings for coronary disease. Many physicians point to Sweden, a country in which people are doing all the dietary, smoking, and exercise maneuvers as are done in the United States, and whose medical facilities are second to none, but whose fatality rate from myocardial infarction is increasing rather than falling. These skeptics comment that although the relationship between the height of the plasma

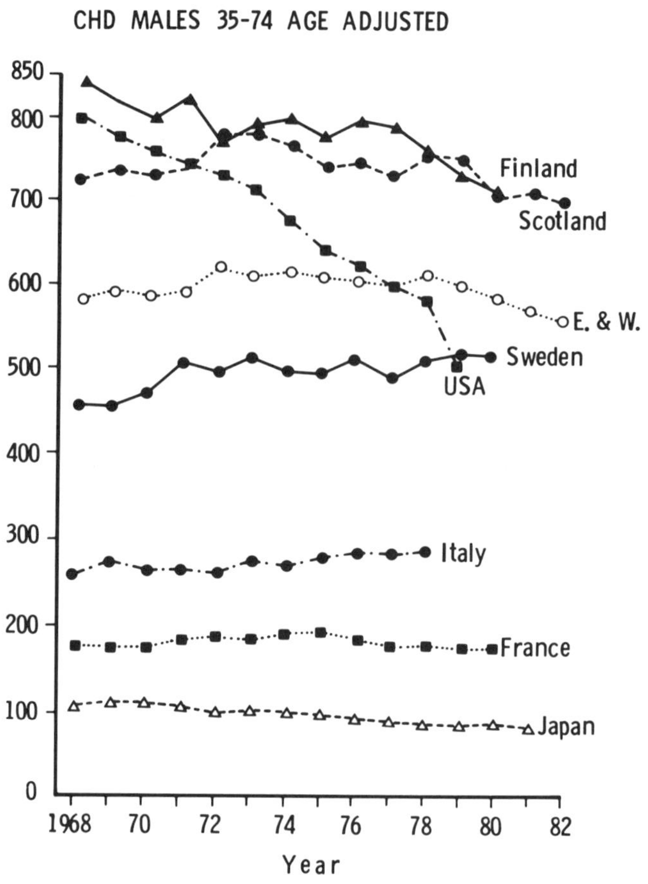

FIGURE 4.1
Coronary Heart Disease Mortality, Males and Females, Aged 35–74, Selected Countries, 1968–1982 (age adjusted rates per 100,000)

Source: M. G. Marmot, "Interpretation of Trends in Coronary Heart Disease," *Acta Medica Scandinavica Supplement* 701 (1985): 58–65.

cholesterol concentration and arterial pressure and the increased risk of coronary disease is undoubted, the corollary, namely that a decrease in cholesterol or blood pressure will reduce risk, is unproven. In analyzing twenty or so trials of the effects of dietary or drug hypocholesterolemic therapy, they note that only the Lipid Research Clinics Primary Prevention Trial produced evidence of benefit, and that was undertaken in a group of males with high-risk plasma cholesterol concentrations in the

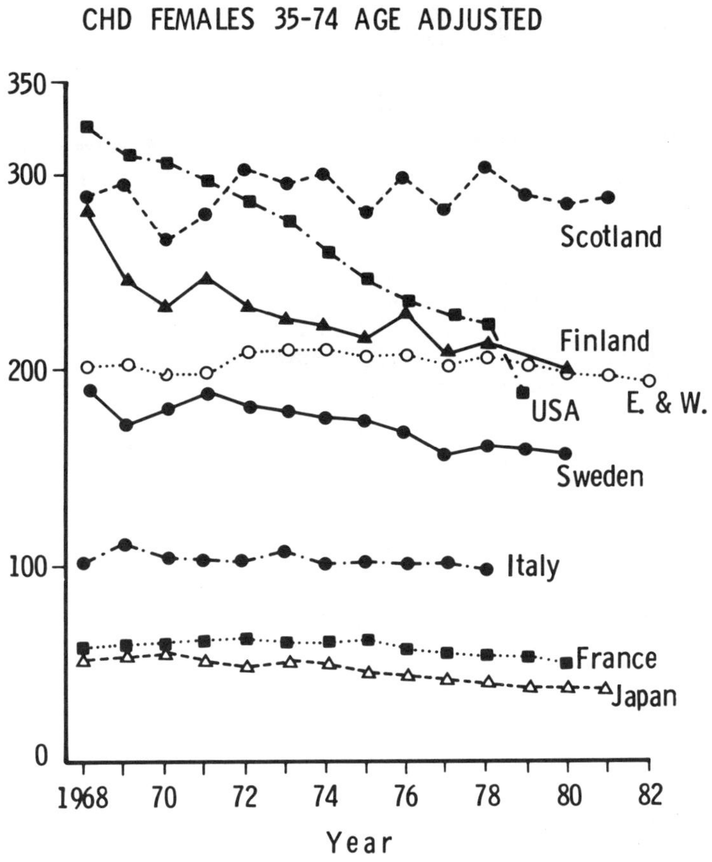

top 5 percent of the distribution curve.[16] To extrapolate from that trial of drug therapy and conclude that dietary maneuvers in subjects with lower cholesterol concentrations will also benefit is not easily justified and to the skeptic, is an inadmissible argument. Peto has pooled the data from all the trials and concluded that protection from coronary disease is provided when plasma cholesterol concentrations are lowered whether by diet or by drugs.[17] The skeptics comment that this decrease in mortality from CAD has been paralleled by an increase in deaths from other causes.

The most recent report on the prevention of coronary disease in the United Kingdom comes from the Working Party of the British Cardiac Society.[18] The report reaches conclusions not very different from its predecessors, although it is less stringent and has more reservation than its U.S. counterparts. The need to prevent or stop cigarette smoking is

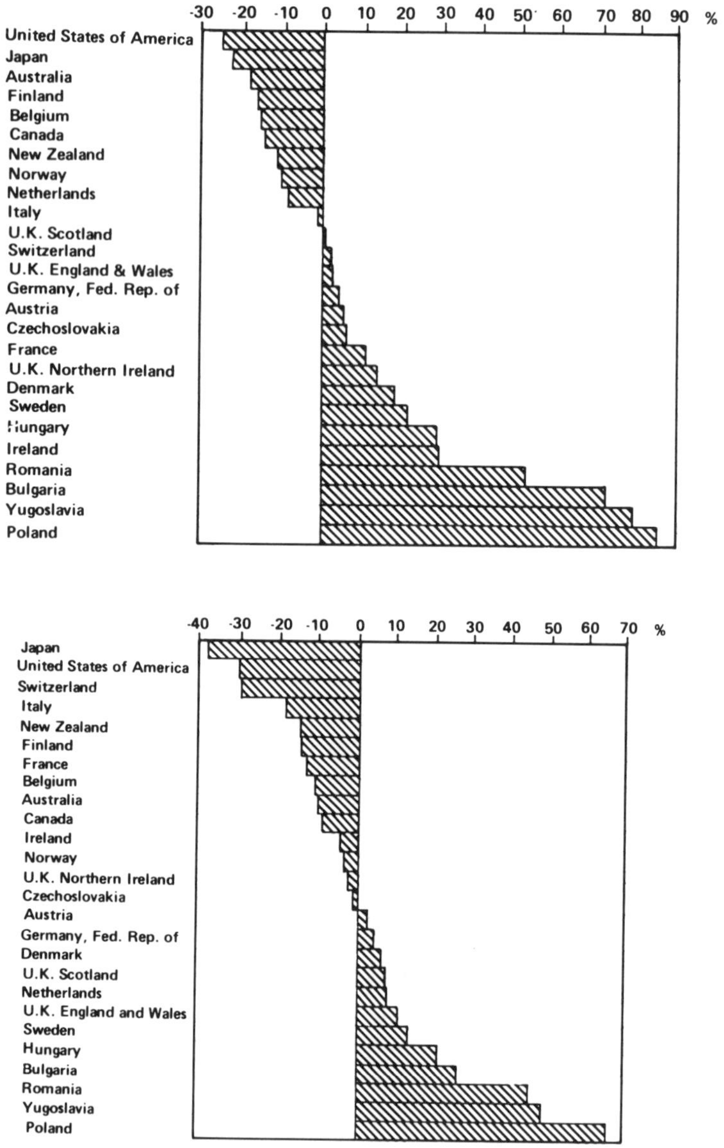

FIGURE 4.2
Average Percentage Change in Mortality from Ischemic Disease, Males and Females, Aged 40–69, Selected Countries, 1968–1979[a]

Note: [a]Based on the slopes of linear regressions fitted to mortality trends in six quinquennial age groups.

Source: M. G. Marmot, "Interpretation of Trends in Coronary Heart Disease," *Acta Medica Scandinavica Supplement* 701 (1985): 58–65.

emphasized. Dietary advice is recommended for those with plasma cholesterol concentrations above 6.5 mmol/l (250 mg/dl), and hypolipidemic drugs are recommended for those with levels over 7.8 mmol/l (300 mg/dl). A "target" cholesterol concentration is set at about 5.2 mmol/1 (200 mg/dl). The report recommends that fat should not form more than 35 percent of energy intake and saturated fat not more than 15 percent. Further, the PS ratio should increase from its present figure of 0.27 to 0.45, the intake of fiber should increase, and of salt should fall.

There are still considerable reservations about this sort of approach among British physicians, although probably to a lesser extent among the public for whom press, radio, and television have urged a turn from the old "unhealthy" to the new "healthy" diet. A recent counter-publication from the Social Affairs Unit in London comprises a contribution from a number of academics, doctors, and nutritionists. In "A Diet of Reason: Sense and Nonsense in the Healthy Eating Debate," they repudiate what they describe as crude and simplistic propaganda about healthy or unhealthy foods and repudiate the evidence for much of the current dietary fashion.[19] A less strident caveat appeared in the British Cardiac Society report: "The recommendations put forward in this report are based on the weight and consistency of the evidence and the likely balance of benefit and harm. They cannot be based on certainty of effectiveness."

Despite conservatism, the scene in Britain is changing slowly. But some British cardiologists will be the last to be converted. In replying to a question about diet by a man in his early forties who had suffered a myocardial infarction and undergone thrombolytic therapy with subsequent angioplasty, a cardiologist replied, "If I knew what to advise about that I would win the Nobel Prize."

Angina Pectoris

Both medical and surgical treatments have a good deal to offer the patient with symptomatic ischemic heart disease, but the proper balance between the two is difficult to ascertain.

The drugs used in medical treatment (beta-adrenergic blocking drugs, calcium entry blockers, and long-acting nitrate preparations) are remarkably effective in relieving symptoms and may also be effective in reducing mortality. For instance, Braunwald has quoted a progressive improvement in annual mortality figures for patients with three-vessel disease treated medically from 11.4 percent in the 1960s, to 4.8 percent in the 1970s, to 3.5 percent in the European Coronary Surgery Study, and 2.1 percent in the Coronary Artery Surgery Study (CASS) which reflects data from the late 1970s.[20] The CASS results were obtained without the probable advantages of the use of calcium entry blockers.[21]

At the same time surgical techniques for coronary artery bypass grafting (CABG) have also improved such that the risk of mortality of the operation has fallen from 5.6 percent in the Veterans Administration (VA) trial published in 1977[22] to 1.4 percent in the CASS series.

Three major trials provide the data that underlie the uncertainty and controversy concerning the role of CABG versus medical treatment. The first of these, the VA study of 1977, concerned a high-risk group with advanced disease. Between 1970 and 1974, 1,015 patients were recruited of whom 13 percent had left main coronary artery disease, 53 percent three-vessel disease, 33 percent two-vessel, and 14 percent one-vessel involvement. Nearly 50 percent combined three-vessel disease with dysfunction of the left ventricle. In contrast to the later CASS and European studies, there was little crossover to surgery of patients originally allocated to medical treatment because of progressive worsening of angina. This trial showed the conclusive superiority of CABG in terms of survival as well as symptomatic relief in patients with left main artery disease, but in other categories no significant difference between medical and surgical treatments emerged. The principal weakness of this study was the high surgical mortality of those early years, 5.6 percent.

The European Coronary Surgery Study and CASS examined quite different cohorts of patients, since at that time it was already recognized that severe angina, unresponsive to medical treatment and left main coronary artery disease required surgery. The results of these two studies are summarized in Figure 4.3 and Table 4.2. Essentially the conclusions most physicians will draw are that surgery has more to offer than medicine in: (1) proximal involvement of the left main coronary artery; (2) patients in whom medical therapy has failed to relieve symptoms (in this situation surgery produces remarkable symptomatic improvement); (3) three-vessel disease, particularly in patients in whom there is dysfunction of the left ventricle, but without infarction.

There is inevitable disquiet among surgeons about these limited conclusions because of the shortcomings of the trials on which they are based.[23] To many cardiac surgeons both the European Study and CASS examine questions only in a highly selected and perhaps unrepresentative group of patients. For instance, CASS included only 37 percent of those initially considered for entry. More importantly, there was a considerable crossover of patients originally allocated to medical treatment to surgery because of worsening angina. The claim is made (and it may be valid) that analysis by intention to treat, although statistically correct, has resulted in an underevaluation of surgical outcome.

Braunwald has referred to the increasing frequency and staggering costs of CABG in the United States. In 1977, 70,000 such operations took place and in 1981, 160,000. Braunwald forecast a slowing or even peaking

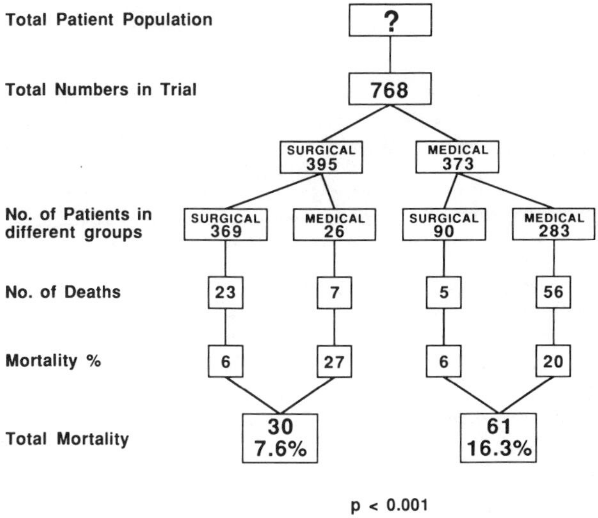

European Coronary Surgery Study (five-year follow-up)

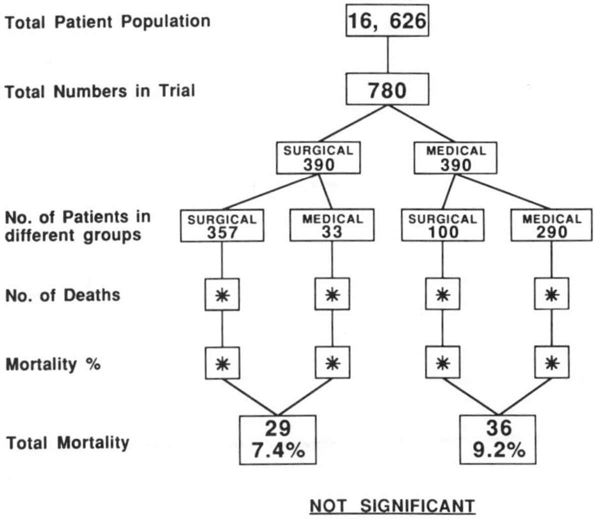

Coronary Artery Surgery Study (CASS)

FIGURE 4.3
European Coronary Surgery Study and Coronary Artery Surgery Study

Source: J. R. Hampton, "Coronary Artery Bypass Grafting for the Reduction of Mortality: An Analysis of the Trials," *British Medical Journal* 289 (1984): 1166–1170.

TABLE 4.2
Data from CASS

	Medical Group	Surgical Group
Overall average annual mortality after 5 years	1.6%	1.5%
Average annual mortality		
Single vessel	1.4	0.7
Two vessels	1.2	1.0
Three vessels	2.1	1.5
Average annual mortality in subgroup with ejection fractions in excess of 50%		
Single vessel	1.1	0.8
Two vessels	0.6	0.8
Three vessels	1.2	1.2

Source: Coronary Artery Surgery Study (CASS) Principal Investigators and Their Associates, "Coronary Artery Surgery Study of Randomized Trial of Coronary Artery Bypass Surgery. Survival Data," *Circulation,* vol. 68 (1983): 939–950.

of these figures when he wrote in 1983, but in 1985 there were 240,000 bypass grafts in the United States [as well as 120,000 percutaneous transluminal coronary angioplasties (PTCA)]. This works out to 1,000 CABG and 502 PTCA per million patients per annum in the United States. The comparable figures for the United Kingdom are 200 per million CABG (against a declared target of 300 per million) and 27 per million angioplasties. The European country with the highest rate of angioplasty is Holland with 189 per million per year, and the overall European figure is currently around 100 per million. In Australia figures for 1985 were 450 per million CABG and 84 per million PTCA; in New Zealand there were 236 per million CABG and 68 per million PTCA.

Are the U.S. figures a reflection of gross overuse of these techniques or do the British reflect gross underuse or both? Almost certainly both for reasons which bear examination.

The first question concerns the likely effects of these surgical approaches on coronary death rates. There are a number of reasons for concluding that the falling death rate from coronary disease in many parts of the world largely reflects a reduced incidence of coronary disease rather than a reduced case fatality rate. The overall changes in the United States are too large to be attributable to the improvement in management of established disease, particularly since the majority of deaths occur out-of-hospital. Changes resulting from improved management would be expected to be selective and most obvious to those who have access to the best medical care, but in fact older blacks are represented in the improved figures that are evident among younger whites. Most convincing, WHO myocardial infarction registers show a high correlation between heart attack rates and mortality from myocardial infarction (Figure 4.4).[24]

A study of myocardial infarction among employees of the Du Pont Company by Pell and Fayerweather supports this conclusion, but it also ascribes a contribution (perhaps some 5 to 25 percent of the total decline) to reduced case fatalities.[25]

If it is accepted that the *incidence* of acute myocardial infarction is falling, it is not possible to decide what contribution comes from changes in life-style (smoking habits, diet, exercise), what from improved drug therapy of symptomatic coronary disease short of infarction, what from CABG or angioplasty, and what from unidentified factors. It is unlikely that medical and surgical treatment play a large part since both are fully

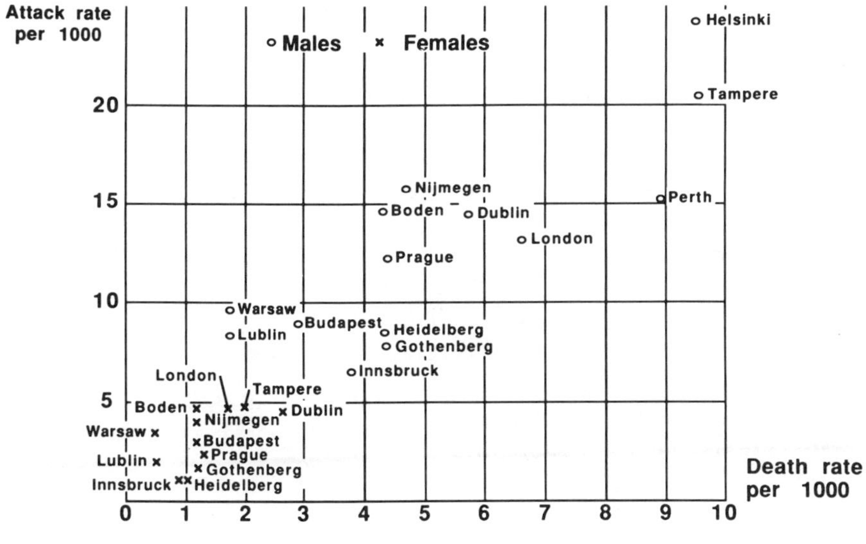

FIGURE 4.4
Correlation Between the Attack Rate of Acute Myocardial Infarction and the Death Rate, Males and Females, Aged 55–64

Note: Attack rate computed from the registers and the death rate from Category 401 of the ICD.

Source: "Public Health in Europe," *Myocardial Infarction Community Register* (Copenhagen: WHO, 1976).

available with a high degree of expertise in Sweden where rates of fatal coronary disease are rising.

The lower rates of bypass grafting and angioplasty in the United Kingdom again may be cultural in a way analogous to population resistance to dietary changes. As Jennett pointed out in 1982, the British distrust technological medicine.[26] The term carries pejorative overtones and in all parts of the world society is increasingly concerned that expensive high-tech procedures are largely responsible for the uncontrolled escalation of health care costs. The emphasis of the central government in Britain now is toward community health and the chronic sector rather than the acute. In considering the specific issue of CABG, Jennett recalls the 1980 finding by an American cardiologist that some threefold more CABG operations were performed by "fee for service" surgeons than by salaried colleagues participating in pre-paid health care plans. In London, too, more such operations are done privately for patients from the Middle East than in the rest of the United Kingdom under the auspices of the National Health Service (NHS).

Another important factor in the much smaller number of operations for coronary disease in Britain is the lack of money and technical resources available to the physicians and surgeons working in the increasingly hard-pressed NHS. Although under Mrs. Thatcher more money is spent on the NHS than ever before, the increase is going to physicians in family practice, to the chronic and long-term psychiatric sector rather than to the acute services, and the teaching hospitals. The United States spends three times as much on health per capita than the United Kingdom, and twice as much per head on hospitalized patients. Henry Aaron and William Schwartz have brought out the stark differences that these overall figures disguise.[27] Per capita again, compared to the United States the United Kingdom has

88 percent as many acute beds
70 percent as many hospital admissions
67 percent as many doctors
50 percent as many radiological investigations with fewer films per examination
33 percent as much maintenance dialysis for renal failure
17 percent of CT scan facilities
5-10 percent of intensive care facilities

How a shortage of resources can be rationalized into clinical decisions to do less dialysis or CABG in the United Kingdom is convincingly described by Aaron and Schwartz. What the "proper" rates for coronary bypass grafting should be no one knows. Whether the MONICA register of incidence, death rates, risk factors, and methods of treatment will ultimately answer this question is quite uncertain; and of course as data are gathered, treatments change.

The most important recent change must be percutaneous transluminal coronary angioplasty (PTCA). PTCA, first reported in 1978, has been undertaken in a relatively small way in the United Kingdom since 1980. No formal trials of angioplasty versus vein grafting or medical treatment have been reported. Despite this, the application of the technique has grown steadily from the dilatation of a single stenosed vessel to multiple vessels, from one proximal lesion to more than one, from patients with stable angina to those with unstable angina and from concentric to eccentric vascular lesions. PTCA is increasingly used after acute myocardial infarction treated successfully by thrombolytic therapy. Complications are not unknown with mortality at approximately 1 percent, iatrogenic myocardial infarction 5 percent, new angina 7 percent, and acute need for vein graft surgery 5-7 percent. Late restenosis may occur in as often as 33 percent of cases and in one recent series overall rates of failure were as high as 27 percent. In this context, much depends on the skill and experience of the physician performing the procedure.[28]

Acute Myocardial Infarction

The management of acute myocardial infarction offers the most alternatives available to the physician. Approaches vary from care at home without hospital admission to the Seattle program of training the general public in techniques of cardiopulmonary resuscitation (CPR) and the provision of superbly efficient paramedic emergency services. Within hospital coronary units there is a bewildering array of possible options in drug therapy with recent emphasis on thrombolysis followed urgently by angiography and, when feasible, angioplasty.

Home Versus Hospital Care

The results of two randomized control trials of hospital versus home care of acute myocardial infarction were published in the United Kingdom in 1976 and 1978.[29] Neither produced an unequivocal result. The Bristol study (1976) randomized only a low risk group with a low mortality in both hospital and home patients, and it consisted of only some 24 percent of those who could have been included. The Nottingham team (1978) sent a mobile coronary care unit to patients' homes but did not randomly allocate home or hospital care until two hours after onset of the first symptom. More than 60 percent of deaths from acute myocardial infarction occur within one hour of the first symptom and, in fact, a recent Belfast series showed a median survival time of only eighty-four minutes, so that the Nottingham results apply to only a fraction of all patients suffering acute infarction. A possible conclusion is that among patients with no complications who have survived the critical first two hours after infarction, there is no evidence that admission to a coronary care unit offers advantages over care at home. There are reservations about even that conclusion since neither study included sufficient numbers to demonstrate small differences in outcome between the two approaches.

Mobile Coronary Care and Resuscitation at Home

Some 30,000 deaths from coronary disease occur outside of hospitals per year in Britain and most of these result from ventricular fibrillation. In the United States this problem has been recognized by the creation of more than 300 local emergency services, each with mobile units and paramedical personnel who have undergone up to 1,600 hours of training in such techniques as defibrillation, intubation, and even the use of emergency drugs. The most successful of these must be the Seattle program in which in a health conscious community more than one-third of the adult population have been trained in cardiopulmonary resuscitation.[30] There is evidence of enviable achievements by the paramedical teams which have genuinely improved out-of-hospital cardiac arrest survival. In 1980, the mean time between collapse of the patient and arrival of the paramedical team was 7.7 minutes. With such a service and in such a community trained in "bystander CPR," survival of arrest to reach the hospital can be achieved in as many as 43 percent of cases.

In Britain the scene is again markedly different. The 1975 report of the British Cardiac Society and the Royal College of Physicians urged the Department of Health to promote the development of units capable of producing mobile coronary care out of the hospital.[31] The department did respond by funding research in this field but concluded in 1976 that "no firm evidence has emerged that the use of specially equipped ambulances manned by ambulance men who have received training in advanced techniques significantly alters the overall mortality rate of patients suffering from acute myocardial infarction."

As Hampton has pointed out, a critical factor in making this a difficult problem in Britain relates to the traditional handling of emergency problems at home by general practitioners and/or by the ambulance service.[32] The trial of the effectiveness of mobile coronary care undertaken in Nottingham illustrates this well. Because of a wish to confine the use of coronary care ambulances and trained crews to likely myocardial infarcts these teams were predominantly called only when the diagnosis had been considered by the family doctor. They therefore tended largely to patients who had survived that critical early hour.

Patients who bypassed their doctors by calling "999" tended to have shorter histories and could have been more suitable for coronary ambulances, but they were handled primarily by the routine ambulance service.

Although at a meeting of interested parties at the Royal Society of Medicine in 1984, a firm recommendation was issued to provide an extensive training program for the public in cardiopulmonary resuscitation in Britain, and the "Save a Life" campaign was launched in October 1986, current political attitudes about the financing of the acute services in the United Kingdom make it unlikely that the scene will change greatly in the foreseeable future.

Coronary Care Unit Management

Coronary care unit management varies among countries and among units within countries. For instance, some 33 percent of patients admitted to units in Italy between 1981 and 1984 were given intravenous nitrates; the figure in Sweden for comparable treatment was 1 percent. Again, in relation to secondary prevention by beta adrenergic blockade, only 5 percent of Danish coronary patients received such treatment compared with 24 percent in the United Kingdom, and 40 percent in Sweden.

Against this background, Drs. Erling Birk Madsen and Paul Ebbe Nielsen have been examining current practice in treating myocardial infarction in Denmark.[33] They have kindly allowed me to quote their data, previously reported to the Danish Society of Internal Medicine and the Danish Society of Cardiology. The survey did not enquire about the use of coronary angiography or angioplasty in the acute phase since these techniques are not widely available in Denmark.

The cooperating hospitals altogether admitted 14,557 patients with acute myocardial infarction in the year of analysis, of whom 4,808 came to small hospitals, 6,689 to county hospitals, and 3,120 to university hospitals. Care was provided largely by general internists in the small hospitals but predominantly by cardiologists in the county and teaching institutions. Information was sought about four broad categories of patients: (1) those with subendocardial infarction, (2) uncomplicated inferior infarction, (3) uncomplicated anterior infarction, and (4) complicated anterior infarction. Table 4.3 shows the variable duration of monitoring, bed rest, hospital stay, and convalescence in these four categories according to the type of hospital to which the patients had been admitted.

Perhaps more surprising is the variable but overall remarkably sparing use of beta adrenergic blocking drugs after infarction (Table 4.4). Recent evidence certainly suggests that these drugs given intravenously

TABLE 4.3
Treatment of Myocardial Infarction by Patient Category and Type of Hospital, Denmark, 1986

	Monitoring Phase (days)	Confined to Bed/Chair (days)	Total Days in Hospital	Convalescence (weeks)
Uncomplicated Subendocardial Infarction				
Smaller hospitals	2–14	1–14	7–21	2–12
County hospitals	1–10	1–8	7–17	3–8
University hospitals	2–14	1–4	7–14	0–7
Uncomplicated Transmural Inferior Infarction				
Smaller hospitals	2–14	1–14	7–22	0–12
County hospitals	3–11	1–11	7–21	3–8
University hospitals	2–7	1–6	7–12	0–8
Uncomplicated Transmural Anterior Infarction				
Smaller hospitals	2–14	1–14	7–22	3–12
County hospitals	3–11	1–14	10–21	3–8
University hospitals	2–12	1–6	7–19	0–8
Transmural Anterior Infarction Complicated by Pulmonary Oedema and Ventricular Arrhythmias				
Smaller hospitals	3–21	1–20	10–28	4–14
County hospitals	5–15	1–12	11–25	3–15
University hospitals	4–16	1–7	11–21	0–12

Note: Cooperating hospitals included 45 smaller hospitals, 24 county hospitals, and 10 university hospitals.

Source: E. B. Madsen and P. E. Nielsen, "Coronary Regimes in Denmark 1986," (personal communication).

TABLE 4.4
Treatment of Acute Myocardial Infarction by Type of Hospital, Denmark, 1986

Is Beta-Adrenergic Blockade Routinely Used Unless Specifically Contraindicated?	Number of Hospitals	
	Yes	No
Smaller hospitals	8	37
County hospitals	4	20
University hospitals	1	9
Total	13 (16%)	66

Are Anticoagulants Used Routinely Unless Specifically Contraindicated?	Yes		
	All Patients	High-Risk Patients	No
Smaller hospitals	3	9	33
County hospitals	1	12	11
University hospitals	3	7	0
Total	7	28	44

Are Exercise ECGs Used Regularly After Recovery?	Yes		
	Before Discharge	At Follow-Up	No
Smaller hospitals	2	6	37
County hospitals	0	4	20
University hospitals	2	2	6
Total	4	12	63

Note: Cooperating hospitals included 45 smaller hospitals, 24 county hospitals, and 10 university hospitals.

Source: E. B. Madsen and P. E. Nielsen, "Coronary Regimes in Denmark 1986," (personal communication).

soon after the onset of symptoms reduce mortality. For instance, 15 mg metoprolol (or placebo) given intravenously to 1,359 patients within twelve hours of the first symptom and continued by mouth for ninety days, reduced mortality by some 36 percent in one study.[34] In another, 16,000 patients were randomly allocated to placebo or to 5-10 mg iv of atenolol within five hours of onset, with oral atenolol for seven days thereafter.[35] There was a 15 percent benefit in survival from active drug treatment. Yusuf et al. have re-examined the twenty-four trials set up to determine the usefulness of less acutely prescribed beta blocking drugs after acute myocardial infarction.[36] Although twenty-one of these twenty-four provided inconclusive results, the aggregated results appropriately weighted suggest a 25 percent benefit from treatment. However, these results, although widely quoted and apparently statistically sound, have not convinced Danish physicians (and many colleagues in other parts of the world) to prescribe beta blockers with any frequency, partly because of the perception that for the individual the advantage of treatment appears slim, particularly in light of the harmful effects to be expected in the event of bradycardia, atrioventricular block, hypotension, or left ventricular failure.

Table 4.4 shows the considerable differences in the use of anticoagulants and a similar degree of variability in the use of post-infarction exercise ECG examinations.

These are only examples from the Danish study which confirms the differences in treatment of acute myocardial infarction. Data about outcomes are not available but will be gathered in due course.

Thrombolytic Therapy

The return to the earlier view that acute myocardial infarction is essentially a thrombotic process has led to a renaissance of concern about clotting and particularly therapeutic fibrinolysis. The available agents are streptokinase, urokinase, and the "targeted" preparations of acylstreptokinase, prourokinase, and recombinant human plasminogen activator. Each of these can be given intravenously or directly into the coronary circulation. The many trials undertaken in the last four to five years in both Europe and the United States have been concerned primarily with rates of recanalization of previously occluded vessels, and the bleeding complications of therapy rather than increased survival or cardiac function. They have been discussed by Sherry in the United States whose views have been echoed by Mitchell in the United Kingdom.[37] The current state of knowledge does not allow firm conclusions about intravenous (simpler, quicker, and perhaps less effective) versus intracoronary administration. Nor does it indicate any clear advantage of the newer recombinant plasminogen activator over acylated streptokinase, prourokinase, or even "straight" streptokinase or urokinase. Bleeding complications occur with all of these agents and all appear capable of recanalizing vessels and salvaging myocardium at risk. To quote Verstraete's summary, reproduced in Mitchell's 1986 review:

> Coronary thrombi can be safely lysed by both coronary and intravenous agents; widespread application of intracoronary thrombolysis is not practical; high dose short duration intravenous treatment produces acceptable reperfusion rates without major bleeding problems and can be applied in

ordinary district hospitals; targeted activators such as recombinant tissue plasminogen activator or acylated streptokinase probably do have advantages but a full comparative appraisal of costs and benefits must await the results of trials.[38]

Overall Conclusion

Cardiovascular diseases remain the commonest cause of morbidity and mortality in the developed world. Huge sums are spent treating established disease, in many situations with no more than the most scanty knowledge of the long-term effect of treatment on outcome. Clinical trials such as the MRC mild hypertension trial or CASS are immensely costly and do not provide the clear guidance the clinician needs. Geoffrey Rose, a most distinguished epidemiologist, has recently concluded that those and other trials have failed to provide "proof" either of etiology or of certainty of preventive measures in cardiovascular diseases.[39] The problems appear bigger and the rewards of such trials smaller than had been anticipated, but they have contributed *something* to knowledge and do provide a slightly firmer foundation on which to make decisions.

Such decisions now depend on judgment rather than proof. What should they be? The biggest problem is undoubtedly coronary artery disease. It is a reasonable conclusion that any form of treatment for established disease is of limited value and that the most practical and sensible approach is to concentrate on *prevention* by changes in diet and life-style, and on etiology, and better definitions of risk to the individual by basic research such as that already begun so successfully in the field of lipid metabolism by Goldstein and Brown.[40] It seems unwise to allow further spending of large sums of money on heroic resuscitation measures for established disease, or larger trials which at best demonstrate the marginal superiority of one treatment over another. But the continued uncontrolled proliferation of new clinical and technological approaches to established coronary artery disease will be hard to prevent unless current attitudes among clinicians change radically in the near future.

Notes

1. See S. J. Pocock, "Current Issues in the Design and Interpretation of Clinical Trials," *British Medical Journal* 290 (1985):39–42; and G. Rose, "Role of Controlled Trials in Evaluating Preventive Medicine Procedures," in *The Value of Preventive Medicine*, Ciba Foundation Symposium 110 (London: Pitman Books Ltd., 1985), pp. 183–201.

2. B. Rajagopalan and J.G.G. Ledingham, "Management of the Hypertensive Crisis," in *Cardiology* 1, edited by P. Sleight and E. Fries (London: Butterworth Scientific, 1982).

3. Hypertension Detection and Follow-up Program (HDFP), "The Effect of Treatment on Mortality in 'Mild' Hypertension: Results of the Hypertension Detection and Follow-up Program," *New England Journal of Medicine* 307 (1982):976–980.

4. C. J. Bulpitt et al., "The Survival of Treated Hypertensive Patients and Their Cause of Death: A Report from the DHSS Hypertensive Care Computing Project," *Journal of Hypertension* 4 (1986): 93–99; and C. G. Isles et al., "Mortality of the Glasgow Blood Pressure Clinic," *Journal of Hypertension* 4 (1986): 141–156.

5. A. V. Chobanian, "Antihypertensive Therapy in Evolution," *New England Journal of Medicine* 314 (1986):1701–1702.

6. E. D. Freis, "Should Mild Hypertension be Treated?" *New England Journal of Medicine* 307 (1982):306–309; A. Breckenridge, "Treating Mild Hypertension," *British Medical Journal* 291 (1985):89–90. Also see D. Hyman and N. M. Kaplan, "Treatment of Patients with Mild Hypertension," *Hypertension* 7 (1985):165–170.

7. Management Committee of the Australian National Blood Pressure Study, "Prognostic Factors in the Treatment of Mild Hypertension," *Circulation* 69 (1984): 668–676; and A. Helgeland, "Treatment of Mild Hypertension, A Five Year Controlled Drug Trial. The Oslo Study," *American Journal of Medicine* 69 (1980):725–732. See also Management Committee, "The Australian Therapeutic Trial in Mild Hypertension," *Lancet* 1 (1980):1261–1267; and Management Committee, "The Australian Therapeutic Trial on Untreated Mild Hypertension," *Lancet* 1 (1982):185–191.

8. Multiple Risk Factor Intervention Trial (MRFIT), "Risk Factor Changes and Mortality Results," *Journal of the American Medical Association* 248 (1982): 1456–1477.

9. Medical Research Council Working Party, "MRC Trial of Mild Hypertension: Principal Results," *British Medical Journal* 291 (1985):97–104. See also O. Paul, "The Medical Research Council Trial," *Hypertension* 8 (1986):733–736.

10. D. E. Grobbee and A. Hofman, "Does Sodium Restriction Lower Blood Pressure?" *British Medical Journal* 293 (1986):27–29.

11. R. Stamler et al., "Nutritional Therapy of High Blood Pressure: Trial Report of a Four-Year Randomised Controlled Trial—The Hypertension Control Program," *Journal of the American Medical Association*, in press.

12. M. G. Marmot, "Interpretation of Trends in Coronary Heart Disease Mortality," *Acta. Med. Scand* (suppl.) 701 (1985):58–65. See also K. Clemura and Z. Pisa, "Recent Trends in Cardiovascular Disease Mortality in 27 Industrialized Countries," *World Health Statistics Quarterly* 38 (1985).

13. *Diet and Coronary Heart Disease. Report of the Advisory Panel of the Committee on Medical Aspects of Food Policy* (London: Her Majesty's Stationary Office, 1974 and 1977; and "Prevention of Coronary Heart Disease. Report of the Joint Working Party of the Royal College of Physicians of London and the British Cardiac Society," *Journal of the Royal College of Physicians*, vol. 10 (1976): 214–274.

14. E. H. Ahrens, "The Diet-heart Question in 1985: Has It Really Been Settled?" *Lancet* 1 (1985):1085–1087; "Britain Needs a Food and Health Policy: The Government Must Face Its Duty," *Lancet* 2 (1986):434–436; Consensus Con-

ference, "Lowering Blood Cholesterol to Prevent Heart Disease," *Journal of the American Medical Association* 253 (1985):2080–2090; AHA Special Report, "Recommendation for the Treatment of Hyperlipidaemia in Adults," *Circulation* 69 (1984):1067A–1090A; and M. F. Oliver, "Consensus on Nonsensus Conferences on Coronary Heart Disease," *Lancet* 1 (1985):1087–1089.

15. A. Yarrow, *Politics, Society and Preventive Medicine* (London: Nuffield Provincial Hospitals Trust, 1986).

16. Lipid Research Clinics Program, "The Lipid Research Clinics Coronary Primary Prevention Trial Results. I. Reduction in Incidence of Coronary Heart Disease," *Journal of the American Medical Association* 251 (1984):351–364.

17. Richard Peto, cited in *The Value of Preventive Medicine,* Ciba Foundation Symposium 110 (London: Pitman Publishing, 1985), p. 77.

18. The British Cardiac Society Working Party on Coronary Prevention, "Conclusions and Recommendations," *British Heart Journal* 57 (1987): 188–189; and *Report of the British Cardiac Society Working Party on Coronary Disease Prevention* (London: British Cardiac Society, 1987).

19. Social Affairs Unit, "A Diet of Reason, Sense and Nonsense in the Healthy Eating Debate" (London: Social Affairs Unit, 1986).

20. E. Braunwald, "Effects of Coronary Artery Bypass Grafting on Survival," *New England Journal of Medicine* 309 (1983):1181–1184.

21. CASS Principal Investigators and Their Associates, "Coronary Artery Surgery Study (CASS) of Randomized Trial of Coronary Artery Bypass Surgery. Survival Data," *Circulation,* vol. 68 (1983): 939–950.

22. Veterans Administration Cooperative Study, "Treatment of Chronic Stable Angina. A Preliminary Report of Survival. Data of the Randomized Veterans Administration Cooperative Study," *Journal of the American Medical Association* 297 (1977):621–627.

23. G. S. Weinstein and B. Levin, "The Coronary Artery Surgery Study (CASS): A Critical Appraisal," *Journal of Thoracic Cardiovascular Surgery* 90 (1985): 541–548. See also R. P. Anderson, "Will the Real CASS Stand Up? A Review and Perspective on the Coronary Artery Surgery Study," *Journal of Thoracic Cardiovascular Surgery* 91 (1986): 698–709.

24. "Public Health in Europe," *Myocardial Infarction Community Register* (Copenhagen: WHO, 1976).

25. S. Pell and M. P. H. Fayerweather, "Trends in the Incidence of Myocardial Infarction and in Associated Mortality and Morbidity in a Large Employed Population 1957-1983," *New England Journal of Medicine* 312 (1985):1005–1011.

26. B. Jennett, *High Technology Medicine: Benefits and Burdens. Rocking Carling Fellowship* (London: Nuffield Provincial Hospitals Trust, 1984).

27. Henry Aaron and William Schwartz, *The Painful Prescription: Rationing of Hospital Care* (Washington, D.C.: Brookings Institution, 1984).

28. C. D. G. Oakley, "Coronary Angioplasty–What Can We Reasonably Expect?" *British Heart Journal* 55 (1986):221–222.

29. J. D. Hill, J. R. Hampton, and J.R.A. Mitchell, "Home or Hospital for Myocardial Infarction: Who Cares?" *American Heart Journal* 98 (1979): 545–547.

30. M. S. Eisenberg, L. Bergner, and A. Hallstrom, "Out of Hospital Cardiac Arrest: Improved Mortality with Paramedic Services," *Lancet* (1980): 812–815.

31. "The Care of the Patient with Coronary Heart Disease. Report of a Joint

Working Party of the Royal College of Physicians of London and the British Cardiac Society," *Journal of the Royal College of Physicians,* vol. 10 (1975): 5–46.

32. J. R. Hampton, "Coronary Patient-Early Treatment," editorial, *British Heart Journal* 46 (1981):117–120.

33. E. B. Madsen and P. E. Nielsen, "Coronary Regimes in Denmark 1986" (personal communication).

34. MIAMI Trial Research Group, "Metoprolol in Acute Myocardial Infarction (MIAMI): A Randomised Placebo-Controlled International Trial," *European Heart Journal* 6 (1985):199–126.

35. ISIS-I (First International Study of Infarct Survival) Collaborative Group, "Randomised Trial of Intravenous Atenolol Among 16,027 Cases of Suspected Acute Myocardial Infarction," *Lancet* 2 (1986):57–66.

36. S. Yusuf et al., "Beta Blockade During and After Myocardial Infarction. An Overview of the Randomised Trials," *Progressive Cardiovascular Disease* 27 (1985):335–371.

37. S. Sherry, "Tissue Plasminogen Activator (tPA). Will It Fulfill Its Promise?" *New England Journal of Medicine* 313 (1985):1014--1017.

38. J. R. A. Mitchell, "Back to the Future. So What *Will* Fibrinolytic Therapy Offer Your Patients with Myocardial Infarction?" *British Medical Journal* 292 (1986):973–978; and "Streptokinase in Acute Myocardial Infarction," *Lancet* 1 (1986):421–422.

39. G. Rose, "Role of Controlled Trials in Evaluating Preventive Medicine Procedures."

40. J. L. Goldstein and M. S. Brown, "LDL Reception and the Regulation of Cellular Cholesterol Metabolism," *Journal of Cellular Science* (supplement) (1985): 131–137.

5

A Catastrophic Disease Perspective on Organ Transplantation

Roger W. Evans

Organ transplants, particularly heart and liver transplants, have often been criticized on the grounds that they are too costly given other health care priorities.[1] It has been argued, for example, that there are many other less costly health interventions to which there is limited access, and that access would be enhanced if the resources allocated to transplantation were diverted to these other worthy interventions. In a similar vein, preventive health care initiatives are often pitted against transplantation as being more cost-effective and more worthy of support than drastic organ transplant procedures.[2] These arguments, of course, have some merit, but decisions as to what constitute appropriate resource allocations are debatable. The simple solutions, such as disease prevention, can be deceiving, as Russell has recently demonstrated.[3] Only the naive person would argue that prevention is *not* a reasonable objective to pursue; however, depending upon the nature and extent of our preventive health care efforts, we must recognize that they, too, can be cost ineffective.

Central to discussions of resource constraints and resource allocation is the underlying concern about the development of consistent health care policy, as I have argued elsewhere.[4] In pursuit of fair and equitable health care policies, it is clear that in retrospect we have already committed major errors in policy formulation, if our ultimate goal is to inculcate and raise a sense of receptivity within the population for preventive health care.[5] Nonetheless, we are somewhat constrained by past decisions, and find it impossible to eschew what are perceived as bad public health care policies.[6] Ultimately it seems our concern about health care costs has served to spur increased interest in preventive health care measures.[7] Despite our cost-containment objectives, it is difficult, for obvious reasons, to turn back the health policy clock by radically altering previous decisions that have substantially increased overall health care expenditures. This, for example, is true with the End-

Stage Renal Disease Program (ESRD)—a $2.2 billion per year program that benefits approximately 85,000 people.[8] It is noteworthy that in 1985 health care expenditures in the United States totaled $425 billion.[9] As a group, ESRD patients accounted for one-half of 1 percent of total health care expenditures. National health expenditures amounted to $1,721 per person in 1985.[10] The average annual expenditure per dialysis patient is in excess of $25,000. While the ESRD Program has been criticized, few have advocated its termination.

Clearly, among the most significant health care issues of the day are those that surround chronic disabling illness, of which the majority of us will die at considerable expense.[11] From an economic viewpoint, heart and liver transplantation nicely illustrates the nature of the problem and serves to underscore the complexity of deciding who will get treated at significant expense to insurers.

The primary objective of this chapter is to put organ transplantation in perspective by examining how catastrophic or high-cost illness has more pervasive implications than most of us recognize. Transplantation underscores the basic health care dilemma that we will increasingly face if our goal is to promote longevity without regard to cost. Only recently have explicit concerns been voiced as to whether much of the catastrophic care that we are capable of providing is cost-effective.

Organ Transplantation: Specific Issues and Research Findings

Before developing a catastrophic disease perspective on organ transplantation, it is important that we understand some key issues and facts specific to transplantation. An economic and policy analysis is certainly deficient if it fails to come to grips conceptually with transplantation as a complicated surgical procedure. Also, the results of reasonably well-grounded empirical research have been ignored by some policy-makers who have chosen to overstate their case, either for or against transplantation.[12] For example, many attempts to analyze the economic consequences of transplantation have erringly focused on the *need* for transplants, rather than the *supply* of donor organs, even though total program expenditures associated with transplantation are determined by the latter.[13]

We also must recognize that transplant candidates have costs associated with their care regardless of whether they receive a transplant.[14] Transplant candidates fall into the more general category of patients dying with a *terminal* condition. They differ from other terminally ill patients in that their end-stage disease is amenable to treatment via a costly procedure, i.e., the transplant.

Finally, we must recognize that transplantation does not constitute a cure. Even transplant recipients with the best prognoses require continuing medical care and, thus, will continue to consume health care resources. In this respect, the transplant recipient can be likened to a patient with a chronic disease in need of continuing medical and, possibly, surgical management. It is also true that the transplant recipient can once again become a terminally ill patient (i.e., the transplant may be rejected).

To further clarify and amplify the foregoing, I will frame the following discussion of transplantation as follows: (1) need and supply estimates, (2) procedure and program costs, and (3) the benefits of transplantation.

Need and Supply

Over the past four years significant attention has been directed to organ transplant technology. This is quite startling when consideration is given to the magnitude of the clinical problems these technologies are intended to treat, given appropriate clinical indications for transplant among potential recipients. For example, each year about 775,000 people die from diseases of the heart, but only between 14,000 and 15,000 may have suitable clinical indications for transplantation and are of an appropriate age (there is much debate as to whether patient age is a clinical or social selection criterion).[15] Moreover, when the most conservative or stringent of patient selection criteria are applied, perhaps only 1,000 to 2,000 people in the United States each year are truly "ideal" heart transplant candidates.[16]

Similar discrepancies exist between crude death rates for kidney and liver disease and conservative clinical criteria for the selection of transplant recipients. Table 5.1, for example, summarizes various estimates we have derived during the course of our research. Clearly a sizable discrepancy exists between the death rates for various diseases and the likelihood that a person dying with such conditions might benefit from a transplant.

Despite the discrepancies identified here, however, considerable expansion could be made in the pool of patients considered reasonable candidates for transplantation. *Patient selection criteria are the key.* If these criteria are relaxed, the potential recipient pool can be expanded substantially. For example, among transplant surgeons reference is frequently made to *absolute* and *relative* contraindications to transplant. Relative contraindications are occasionally ignored when selecting transplant candidates. Age is often considered a relative contraindication, as is the presence of some comorbid condition such as diabetes.[17] Over time, as transplant technology improves, various relative contraindications will be eliminated and perhaps what were previously thought of as absolute contraindications will become relative. In short, the number of

TABLE 5.1
Need for Organ Transplant Procedures in the United States

Procedure	Deaths by Disease	Need Estimate[d]	
		Gross Estimate	Refined Estimate
Kidney[a]	22,560	8,500	8,500
Heart[b]	775,248	15,000	2,000
Liver[c]	26,770	9,500	2,300

Notes: [a]Includes nephritis, nephrotic syndrome, and nephrosis.
[b]Includes diseases of the heart only.
[c]Includes chronic liver disease and cirrhosis.
[d]Determined by patient selection criteria.

Source: Data for kidney procedures from National Task Force on Organ Transplantation, *Final Report* (Rockville, Md.: Health Resources and Services Administration, 1986); and National Center for Health Statistics, "Annual Summary of Births, Marriages, Divorces, and Deaths: United States, 1985," *Monthly Vital Statistics Report* 34 (1986): 1–28. Data for heart procedures from R. W. Evans et al., "Donor Availability as the Primary Determinant of the Future of Heart Transplantation," *Journal of the American Medical Association* 225 (1986): 1892–1898; and National Center for Health Statistics, "Annual Summary of Births, Marriages, Divorces, and Deaths: United States, 1985," *Monthly Vital Statistics Report* 34 (1986):1–28. Data for liver procedures from National Center for Health Statistics, "Annual Summary of Births, Marriages, Divorces, and Deaths: United States, 1985," *Monthly Vital Statistics Report* 34 (1986): 1–28; and R. W. Evans, *The Need for and Cost of Liver Transplantation in the U.S. Update Report No. 38, National Kidney Dialysis and Kidney Transplantation Study* (Seattle: Battelle Human Affairs Research Centers, 1984).

people who may benefit from a transplant is determined by the criteria used to select patients. Increasingly liberal criteria will add substantially to the pool of potential transplant recipients. Nonetheless, crude death data are likely to continue to overstate the need for transplantation since few people are likely to become truly appropriate candidates for transplantation.

This brings us to another essential point—the availability of donor organs.[18] As noted above, we can transplant only as many people as we have donor organs. Table 5.2 shows annual estimates of the number of organ donors in the United States.[19] Since kidneys are a paired organ, each donor can potentially be the source of two grafts. This, of course, is not true of either hearts or livers. Moreover, the criteria for selecting heart donors are extremely stringent, while those for liver donors are similar to those for kidneys. In the National Heart Transplantation Study, for example, we estimated that between 15 and 40 percent of all cadaveric kidney donors could potentially serve as heart donors.[20] Recently the annual supply of donor hearts was estimated somewhere between 500 and 1,300. Elsewhere, we have conservatively estimated that about 1,800 livers may currently be available for transplant, although the actual number is probably much higher.[21] Nearly every kidney procured in the United States today is transplanted here or abroad, although at one time it was estimated that there was a wastage or nonviability rate of about 20 percent.[22] In the last year it appears that the nonviability rate has dropped to around 5 percent, which is probably a result of better coordination of efforts to procure donor organs.

As is true of the need for transplantation, the availability of donor organs is determined by selection criteria. If these criteria are relaxed, as some have argued they should be, there could be a substantial increase in donor supply. For example, presently men over the age of thirty-five and women over the age of forty are not considered candidates for heart donation.[23] It is generally believed that heart disease has onset at about these ages. Once again, such criteria can be considered absolute or relative and the specific interpretation of these criteria is subject to variation among transplant teams. Therefore, organ procurement coordinators may check with several transplant teams before they decide that a particular organ, most often a heart, cannot be used.

There are other factors that may narrow the gap between the need for and the supply of organs. They include: (1) better preservation tech-

TABLE 5.2
Estimates of the Number of Organ Donors in the United States, 1980–1985

Year	Total
1980	2,138
1981	2,142
1982	2,300
1983	2,705
1984	3,290
1985[a]	3,637

Note: [a] Estimated from 1985 data published in 1986 by the Health Care Financing Administration.

Source: National Task Force on Organ Transplantation, *Final Report* (Rockville, Md.: Health Resources and Services Administration, 1986).

niques, (2) mechanical replacement organs, and (3) xenografting. I will briefly comment on each of these.

First, organ preservation is a persistent problem. Organs can be preserved outside the body for only relatively short periods of time—kidneys for up to seventy-two hours, hearts for approximately four hours, and livers for approximately twelve hours. Therefore, if a suitable recipient is not near, a perfectly good organ may be wasted. This problem is becoming less of a concern as there has been a marked proliferation of transplant programs throughout the entire United States.[24] Despite the diminished possibility of wastage attributable to the proliferation of transplant programs, advances have been made in cryobiology that may eventually make long-term organ preservation by freezing a reality.[25] Also, perfusion techniques have been developed whereby organs receive adequate supplies of oxygenated blood to prolong their preservation time.

Artificial organs, with the exception of the artificial kidney or dialysis machine, and variations of peritoneal dialysis, have had limited application, and have been exclusive to the heart. A variety of artificial hearts and ventricular assist systems, collectively referred to as mechanical circulatory support systems (MCSSs), are currently available and, with the exception of the Humana Hospital in Louisville, are used solely to bridge patients to transplant.[26] If a viable mechanical heart or assist device can be developed for permanent implantation, the need for such devices could potentially be met. In fact, were this to happen, the constraint may be on the number of qualified teams available to implant them.[27] At any rate, a mechanical substitute or permanent assist device to replace or assist the ailing heart is unlikely to be available within the next five years.[28] No mechanical substitute is available for the liver, although, because of the organ's regenerative properties, attempts have been made to segment a single liver for use on several recipients.

Finally, the functions of the pancreas are currently being supplemented or replaced through the use of insulin pumps.[29] Typically, patients with severe diabetes have depended upon intramuscular insulin injections. The insulin pump permits a more measured administration of insulin, depending upon the need of the particular patient. It is likely that insulin pumps will be used on a much wider scale in the future, and that pancreatic transplantation will continue to have a somewhat limited role for some time.

Xenografting, or the transplantation of organs from other species into humans, holds some promise but is not widely practiced at this time.[30] While xenografts have been performed on several occasions, most recently at Loma Linda University Medical Center (Baby Fae), there are relatively few transplant teams which aspire to perfect this technique.[31]

It is noteworthy, however, that the cardiac transplant team at Columbia Presbyterian Medical Center in New York has recently asked its institutional review board to approve the use of chimpanzee hearts to bridge patients until donor hearts become available. It is likely that xenografting will continue to be the subject of research and that the actual application of the technique will be limited.

The picture that emerges is clear. The gap between the need for donor organs and their availability will be affected by increasing the supply of human organ donors.[32] Recent attempts have been made by individual states through passage of routine inquiry or required request legislation to do this,[33] and, at the federal level an attempt has been made to impose routine inquiry on all states by mandating that hospitals receiving Medicare funds have such a policy in place. Unfortunately, the effect of such policies on organ donation has yet to be evaluated empirically, although preliminary evidence appears to be favorable.

On the downside, a variety of initiatives at the federal, state, and local levels can conceivably have, if they have not already had, a dampening effect on organ donation.[34] The situation has been complicated by the introduction of seat belt laws,[35] laws requiring the use of child-restraint seats,[36] the 55-mph speed limit, drunk driving laws, handgun laws, motorcycle helmet laws, and more proficient trauma care, all of which in principle would reduce donor supply. Improvements in the provision of mental health services would have a similar effect on the incidence of suicide. Therefore, I remain only cautiously optimistic about a sizable increase in the donor pool, despite routine inquiry legislation and efforts to educate the public and medical professionals about the need for donor organs.

Procedure and Program Costs

At the most elementary level, an analysis of the costs of transplantation should distinguish between procedure costs and program costs.[37] Procedure costs refer to the expenditures associated with performing a single transplant, whereas program costs refer to the economic liability a payer incurs when offering coverage for a given procedure or medical service. For example, over the course of one year, a private insurance company may pay for six heart transplants. The cost of treating and caring for these six patients, plus administrative costs, would equal the insurer's total program expenditures. From a payer's perspective, therefore, the total economic impact of transplantation is evaluated in terms of program expenditures, not individual procedure costs. Also, it is noteworthy that while transplant procedure costs may be high, overall program expenditures incurred by an insurer may be viewed as low, in light of the total beneficiary population over which these costs are distributed.

In this regard, it is my hypothesis that when the benefits of a clinical procedure are in doubt (experiment versus therapy) and when considerable controversy has been engendered, the insurer will choose to pay for the procedure if total program costs are expected to be negligible or at least have minimal impact. In short, it is easier to pay than to argue and possibly create a negative public image. Insurers, particularly in the private sector, are sensitive to this because lost enrollees translate into higher beneficiary premiums and higher operating costs. On the positive side, it appears that transplantation has created a new level of beneficiary awareness. People now ask questions about coverage, a matter that heretofore has been largely ignored.

Another distinction that is important in principle but frequently ignored in practice, is that between *costs* and *charges*.[38] Charges are reflected by the patient's hospital bill. They are what the patient, third-party payer, or combination of both is billed for medical care. Costs are expenses the provider actually incurs in providing a good or service, less "profit" which is reflected in the hospital bill. Some payers, such as Medicare, pay neither charges nor actual hospital costs. They may pay more than true costs, but less than actual charges. For example, prior to prospective payment, Medicare paid approximately 80 percent of charges, yielding what was commonly referred to as "Medicare costs."

In assessing the cost of a transplant procedure one must consider the transplant as having several distinct cost components: pretransplant, evaluation and screening, candidacy, transplant, and posttransplant costs. Pretransplant costs are incurred in caring for a patient prior to transplant. Evaluation and screening costs are associated with "working-up" a patient to determine if he or she is a suitable transplant candidate. Candidacy costs are incurred by a patient immediately following acceptance as a transplant candidate through the period immediately before the transplantation. Transplant costs are accumulated from surgery to initial discharge. Finally, postoperative costs are usually summarized according to year since transplant. The major problem with post-transplant costs is determining which are related and unrelated to the transplant per se.

To determine the cost-effectiveness of a given transplant procedure, we must cost out some form of alternative care. This would consist of the cost of the alternative care the patient would have received had the transplant not been performed. The next requirement is to identify a group of patients who receive such treatment. Transplant recipients would be compared with this group. Identifying such a group of patients is not as simple as it might first appear. Upon close examination, it would appear that only those patients who have been declared candidates for the transplant procedure should be compared. This group of patients

TABLE 5.3
Patient Groups and Measures Relevant to Cost-Effectiveness of Organ Transplantation

Nonrecipients	Transplant Recipients
Cost Components	Cost Components
Pretransplant costs	Pretransplant costs
Evaluation costs	Evaluation costs
Candidacy costs	Candidacy costs
	Transplant costs
	Posttransplant costs
Effectiveness	Effectiveness
Patient died	Patient alive
No quality of life	Reasonable quality of life

Source: R. W. Evans, "Cost Effectiveness Analysis of Transplantation," *Surgical Clinics of North America* 66 (1986):603–616.

can be divided into recipients and nonrecipients. The nonrecipients are those patients who did not receive a transplant because a donor organ was not available and who died as a consequence. Therefore, the cost of the alternative treatment would equal the costs incurred by the nonrecipients. But even this comparison is complicated. Table 5.3 reveals the relevant cost components and appropriate effectiveness measures. One assumes equivalence of the two patient groups in terms of both pretransplant, evaluation, and screening costs. They clearly differ with regard to candidacy costs, transplant costs, and posttransplant costs. Neither of the last two components is relevant for nonrecipients. Thus, it would appear that with regard to cost, nonrecipients incur lower costs than recipients. Nevertheless, the critical difference occurs on the effectiveness side of the equation. The nonrecipients died while the majority of recipients are likely to live. In principle it could be argued that the transplant recipients who died should be combined with the nonrecipients to evaluate cost-effectiveness. However, this introduces a different question for analysis—namely, how cost-effective is a failed transplant when compared with one that works? The answer to this question is obvious. If the goal of the transplant is to save a life, the death of a transplant recipient cannot be judged cost-effective.

Table 5.4 summarizes high, low, and average estimates of the charges associated with a variety of transplants. Where available, an estimate of

TABLE 5.4
Estimated Charges Associated with Various Solid Organ Transplant Procedures

Organ	Low	High	Average	Cost per Year of Life Gained
Heart	$57,000	$110,000	$ 95,000	$23,500
Kidney	25,000	45,000	35,000	14,250
Liver	68,000	238,000	130,000	38,000
Pancreas	18,000	50,000	35,000	14,250

Note: Charges are total first-year charges including immunosuppressive drugs.

Source: R. W. Evans, "The Socioeconomics of Organ Transplantation," *Transplantation Proceedings* 17 (supplement) (1985):129–136.

the cost per year of additional life has also been noted. This figure takes into account the expected survival of the patient and distributes the total costs for the care of the patient over this period. Certainly these estimates are highly speculative.

Mentioned previously is the need to cost out the care of the end-stage patient who does not receive a transplant. In the case of the patient with end-stage cardiac disease, we have estimated that as much as $6,000 per month could easily be spent, probably more.[39] Others have attempted to estimate the cost of treating end-stage hepatic disease in the absence of a transplant. For example, O'Donnell and associates found that the cost of medical and surgical therapy for patients with acute variceal bleeding averages $35,000 per case.[40] This estimate is problematic, however, since the patients studied were not considered candidates for liver transplants. The alternative cost of not performing a kidney transplant would be equivalent to the cost of maintenance dialysis, which on average costs about $25,000 per patient annually.

Clearly, end-stage disease can be expensive to treat depending on how aggressively the medical team pursues treatment. Treatment cost is certainly positively correlated with the intensiveness or level of care administered. In the National Heart Transplantation Study we found that, even among transplant recipients, at some institutions patients who died had higher transplant costs than patients who survived.[41] All of this, of course, brings up a related issue, namely the cost of caring for dying patients. Lubitz and Prihoda have shown that 5.9 percent of Medicare beneficiaries who died in 1978 accounted for 27.9 percent of all Medicare expenditures.[42] In the same study, it was also shown that 30 percent of all expenses of decedents occurred in the last thirty days of life, 46 percent in the last sixty days, and 77 percent in the last six months of life.[43] Clearly, dying is costly.[44]

Thus, we begin to see that it is inappropriate to judge the cost of a transplant procedure without relating it to the cost of otherwise treating the end-stage patient in the absence of the transplant. In order to gain perspective on this subject, the costs associated with the routine care of a dying patient must be considered, but even then, much remains to be done if transplantation costs are to be properly accounted and tabulated.

To conclude this discussion, a few comments and estimates concerning program costs and expenditures are in order. Very crude estimates of program expenditures can be derived by multiplying the number of donor organs by the appropriate average cost per transplant for any given year and including the costs associated with the care of transplant recipients from previous years.

Program expenditure data for the treatment of end-stage renal disease in the United States are maintained by the Health Care Financing Administration. With few exceptions, all patients receiving kidney transplants and routine maintenance dialysis in the United States are Medicare-eligible. Dialysis patients are eligible for benefits indefinitely, while transplant recipients have their eligibility discontinued three years after their transplant, provided the graft is retained over this period.

Program expenditure data for dialysis and transplant patients are not reported separately. The data presented in Table 5.5., therefore, reflect total ESRD program expenditures. Kidney transplantation is generally believed to have a clinical outcome superior to that of maintenance dialysis and offers patients a higher quality of life at a considerably lower cost.[45] Many studies have shown that despite the high initial costs, the long-term costs of transplantation are far below those of dialysis.[46]

As shown in Table 5.6, the number of kidney transplants performed per year has continued to increase, with very sizable increases each year beginning in 1982. As described by Eggers, this increase in transplants has had some impact on total Medicare expenditures for renal diseases by slowing overall rates of growth. It is estimated that patients with functioning grafts generate costs that are roughly one-third as great as dialysis patients. Eggers concludes that ". . . as the distribution of the Medicare ESRD population continues to shift toward functioning graft patients, program expenditures will be proportionately attenuated."[47]

Only in June 1986 did Medicare announce coverage of heart transplants for very selected patients. As of yet, Medicare has not actually begun to cover heart transplants. However, in announcing its coverage decision, the Department of Health and Human Services (DHHS) provided estimates of program expenditures likely to be associated with coverage. For example, DHHS estimated that up to ten transplant cen-

TABLE 5.5
Reimbursement Made by the Medicare Program for Services Provided to ESRD Patients Through June 30, 1986 (in millions of dollars)

Type of Payment	1981	1982	1983	1984	1985
Inpatient	$435.0	$518.1	$621.4	$710.1	$709.8
Outpatient	732.5	782.0	854.2	843.9	729.2
Physician/supplier	303.3	354.3	408.1	387.0	425.0
Home health/skilled nursing facility	5.4	6.5	9.9	12.5	11.6
Total	$1,476.2	$1,660.9	$1,893.6	$1,953.5	$1,875.6

Source: End-Stage Renal Disease Program Highlights, 1985 (Baltimore: Health Care Financing Administration, 1986).

ters would qualify to perform heart transplants and that up to sixty-five transplants would be covered by Medicare at a first-year cost of about $5 million.[48] By the time the program has been in operation for five years, it is projected that Medicare will be paying for about 143 transplants a year, costing some $25 million. These estimates include initial transplant costs as well as maintenance costs associated with beneficiaries who already had heart transplants earlier in the program and an inflation factor.

Medicare covers liver transplants for an *extremely* selective group of patients—children eighteen-years of age or younger with biliary atresia or other rare congenital anomalies. In fact, since Medicare's decision was announced in 1984, not a single liver transplant has been paid for under the program.

Thus far this discussion of program expenditures has been limited to a single insurer—Medicare. Obviously, Medicare is not the only health insurance program concerned about expenditures. In fact, all payers—Medicaid plans, private insurers, health maintenance and preferred provider organizations—have concerns about program expenditures.[49] Unfortunately, it is difficult to assess the likely impact that transplantation will have on each insurer or type of insurer. In only one instance did the National Task Force on Organ Transplantation attempt to derive program expenditures according to a major category of payer.[50] This was done for a public payer that would assume responsibility for patients who lacked coverage for a heart or liver transplant. The task force report estimated, for example, that 64 million people did not have coverage for a heart transplant and that 61 million did not have coverage for a liver transplant.

This concludes our very brief discussion of program expenditures. As argued previously, although transplant procedure costs are quite high, total program expenditures a given payer may incur are often likely to be quite low, given the current availability of donor organs. This situation is likely to change if donor organs become more abundant and patient selection criteria are relaxed.

Benefits of Transplantation

Traditionally when the benefits of transplantation have been discussed, attention has been limited to patient survival and to some extent the vocational rehabilitation of patients.[51] Considerable data on the survival of transplant recipients have now been accumulated and it is clear that heart, kidney, bone marrow, and selected liver transplant recipients enjoy prolonged lives that otherwise would have been impossible. Table 5.7 provides a compilation of the survival rates associated with various organ transplants.[52] With the introduction of new immunosuppressive drugs and techniques many survival rates have improved dramatically. For example, it is now estimated that well over 80 percent of all heart transplant recipients will live one year, over 50 percent five years, and better than 25 percent ten or more years. It is also noteworthy that many

TABLE 5.6
Number of Kidney Transplants Performed by Year, 1973–1985

Year	Number of Transplants
1973	3,017
1974	3,190
1975	3,730
1976	3,504
1977	3,973
1978	3,949
1979	4,271
1980	4,697
1981	4,885
1982	5,358
1983	6,112
1984	6,968
1985	7,695

Source: P. W. Eggers, "Impact of Transplantation on the Medicare ESRD Program," in press.

TABLE 5.7
Transplant Survival Rates

Transplant Procedure	One-Year Patient Survival	One-Year Graft Survival
Kidney	92–95%	71% (cadaver) 88% (living related donor)
Heart	75–85%	
Liver	60–70%	

Source: National Task Force on Organ Transplantation, *Final Report* (Rockville, Md.: Health Resources and Services Administration, 1986).

transplant teams have achieved survival rates that exceed those shown in Table 5.7, underscoring the fact that there is considerable variation across transplant centers not depicted in Table 5.7.

Frequently neglected in the evaluation of organ transplant procedures has been an empirical assessment of the rehabilitation and quality of life of transplant recipients.[53] The quality of life concept is indeed an important one and should, routinely, be the subject of systematic study. Offering a patient extended life without reasonable quality can no longer be considered acceptable.

Elsewhere we have argued that quality of life has both objective and subjective dimensions.[54] Objective indicators include functional ability, ability to work, and health status. Subjective indicators include well-being, psychological affect, and life satisfaction. In both the National Heart Transplantation Study and the National Kidney Dialysis and Kidney Transplantation Study, we studied quality of life intensively. Our results as they apply to heart and kidney transplantation as well as kidney dialysis are shown in Table 5.8. As shown, heart and kidney transplant patients enjoy a similar quality of life. Differences between the two groups are most likely partly due to differences in patient case-mix. For example, the average age of a heart transplant recipient is forty-two while that of a renal transplant recipient is thirty-seven. However, if case-mix adjustments were made statistically, it is likely that the quality of life scores for heart transplant recipients shown in Table 5.8 would be higher.

Also shown in Table 5.8 are the scores on the subjective quality of life indicators for the general population. Clearly transplant recipients compare very well. However, on the objective measures such as health status, neither transplant recipients nor dialysis patients compare well.

TABLE 5.8
Summary of Quality of Life Scores for Heart Transplant, Kidney Transplant, and Kidney Dialysis Patients

Patient Group		Functional Impairment[a]	Ability to Work[b]	Health Status[c]	Well-being[d]	Psychological Affect[e]	Life Satisfaction[f]
Heart							
Transplant	X	1.47	57.88	9.60	11.11	5.49	5.11
Recipient	SD	(.772)	(49.55)	(9.01)	(2.53)	(1.32)	(1.28)
Kidney							
Transplant	X	1.96	74.13	5.52	11.83	5.62	
Recipient	SD	(1.30)	(43.95)	(7.06)	(2.72)	(1.25)	(5.66)
All dialysis	X	2.88	44.68	12.16	10.94	5.27	5.16
patients	SD	(1.43)	(49.75)	(10.54)	(2.72)	(1.26)	(1.64)
General	X	N/A	N/A	N/A	11.77	5.68	5.45
population	SD	N/A	N/A	N/A	(2.21)	(1.12)	(1.25)

Notes: [a]Based on the Karnofsky Index, range of values = 1.0–10.0, where 1.0 = absence of dysfunction and 10 = maximum dysfunction (death).
[b]Ability to work, range of values = 0.0–100.0, where 0.0 = patients unable and 100.00 = patients able.
[c]Total Sickness Impact Profile score only, range of values = 0.0–100.0. Lower scores indicate better health status.
[d]Range of values = 2.1–14.7, where high score = positive well-being.
[e]Range of values = 1.0 to 7.0, where 7.0 = positive effect.
[f]Range of values = 1.0–7.0, where 7.0 = positive satisfaction.
N/A = not available.
X = mean; SD = standard deviation.

Sources: R. W. Evans et al., *The National Heart Transplantation Study: Final Report, Volumes 1–5* (Seattle: Battelle Human Affairs Research Centers, 1984); R. W. Evans et al., *The Treatment of End-Stage Renal Disease in the U.S.: Selected Findings from the National Kidney Dialysis and Kidney Transplantation Study* (Baltimore: Health Care Financing Administration, in press).

These results pose an interesting dilemma. How do we choose to define quality of life? Our intent here is not to resolve this dilemma but, once again, only to show that a procedure whose therapeutic status is in question—such as heart transplantation in recent years—has seemingly achieved status similar to that of kidney transplantation and exceeds that of kidney dialysis.

The Definition of Catastrophic Illness

The preceding discussion makes it impossible for us to ignore the onerous problems accompanying the treatment of catastrophic disease. The costs associated with individual procedures are high and the conditions which patients present for treatment are devastating. It is thus surprising that much of the debate surrounding organ transplantation over the past four years has avoided direct confrontation of this overpowering issue. To better come to grips with the problem, it is important to first consider various definitions of catastrophic illness.

Many definitions of catastrophic illness have been offered and have been reviewed by Berki and associates.[55] They note, for example, that some researchers have adopted a catastrophic threshold approach wherein the focus of attention is a dollar amount expended for health care over a period of time, usually a year. Exemplifying this approach is the work by Schroeder et al. who studied patients who had yearly hospital charges in excess of $4,000 in 1976.[56] A similar approach was followed by Kobrinski and Matteson who examined hospital discharges where total charges, excluding attending physician and surgeon fees, exceeded $4,000 in 1977.[57] Other studies, such as those by Birnbaum, have examined several thresholds including expenditures in excess of $5,000 per calendar year as well as $3,000 per year.[58] Finally, a 1982 Congressional Budget Office (CBO) report looked at several yearly expenditure threshold levels—$3,000, $5,000, $10,000, and $20,000.[59] In addition, the CBO report looked at expenditures accumulated over several consecutive years.

Another approach to defining catastrophic illness relates health care expenditures to total family income which recognizes that catastrophic illness may take on different definitions depending upon the economic resources families command. One CBO report defined an illness as catastrophic when out-of-pocket health expenses exceeded 15 percent of family income.[60]

Other studies have used both threshold levels and family income as the basis upon which to define catastrophic illness. For example, Forthofer et al. used several expenditure thresholds—$1,000, $2,500, and $5,000—and two income-related definitions—expenditures greater than

15 percent of family income and expenditures greater than 50 percent of per capita income.[61]

Berki et al. conclude that ". . . definitions based on family income are generally acknowledged as the most appropriate and meaningful."[62] They indicate that "most" of the state-enacted catastrophic illness programs rely on income-based criteria. However, they also point out that ". . . conventional health insurance does not generally tie benefits to a person's or a family's income level, and therefore any catastrophic coverage that would be provided by insurance companies is quite likely to be defined in terms of set levels of expenditures."

Obviously no single generally accepted definition of catastrophic illness has emerged. This prompted Berki et al. to argue that definitions will vary according to the perspective one adopts, ". . . each characterized by the type of cost considered and the time span during which the accumulation of these costs is observed."[63] These four perspectives, the key elements of which are identified in Table 5.9, are as follows: (1) the social perspective, (2) the individual and family perspective, (3) the perspective of the third-party payer, and (4) the institutional perspective.

As shown in Table 5.9, each of these perspectives focuses on catastrophic illness as a short-term episodic event. This is clearly a deficiency

TABLE 5.9
Definition of Catastrophic Medical Expenses: Key Elements and Perspectives

Perspective	Inclusive of Costs	Unit of Observation and Time Span
Social	All costs direct indirect	Episodes of illness
Individual and family	Out-of-pocket costs actual amount as % of income	Episode for individual for family
Third-party payer	Cost of covered benefits	One-year or other benefit period
Institutional	Reimbursable costs and charges	Discharge

Source: S. E. Berki et al., *High Cost Illness Among Hospitalized Patients. Final Report on Phase I of Contract No. 233-81-3021* (Springfield, Il.: National Technical Information Service, December 1983), p. 11.

that Berki et al. tried to address by examining data for the same people over a three-year period. Unfortunately, data were unavailable on family income which forced Berki et al. to limit their study to an analysis of the institutional perspective and that of third-party payers.[64]

Regardless of the definition adopted, organ transplantation implies a catastrophic disease, both in terms of annual treatment expenditures and percentage of total household income required to pay for treatment. This is particularly true of patients who receive heart or liver transplants, since these are the two most costly transplant procedures generally accepted as therapeutic. Even more startling is the fact that the annual cost of immunosuppressive drugs, required by virtually all transplant recipients, is between $1,000 and $6,000. The most costly of these drugs is cyclosporine which on average costs the patient or a third-party payer between $5,000 and $6,000 per year.[65] This, of course, is atypical of the average person who is likely to have an annual drug expenditure of less than $108.[66]

Of the perspectives presented in Table 5.9, the examination of organ transplantation has largely been limited to that of the third-party payer, with a few casual attempts to apply an institutional perspective. Unfortunately, neither the social perspective nor that of the individual and family has received any systematic and concerted attention. This situation may change, however, as we gain greater familiarity with the long-term consequences of organ transplantation. As noted previously, transplantation is not a cure—the transplant recipient remains a chronically ill person with a rather disconcerting probability of becoming terminally ill should the transplanted organ be rejected. Thus, catastrophic disease may be chronic as well as terminal, and the total cost of catastrophic disease therefore should reflect expenditures during both phases of the patient's illness. Nearly everyone, including transplant recipients, will incur health care costs associated with their death. In a real sense, transplantation merely forestalls the inevitable. With respect to the cost of dying, the issue becomes, do the costs of dying incurred by transplant recipients exceed those of patients who die with conditions for which transplantation is appropriately indicated? If they do, then we can effectively conclude that transplantation adds substantially to the cost of terminal catastrophic illness.

Conceptualization of Costs

In examining and conceptualizing the financial implications of disease and illness, economists often distinguish between *economic costs* and *social costs*.[67] Economic costs are divided into two categories—direct costs and indirect costs. Direct costs, as shown in Figure 5.1, include

FIGURE 5.1 Conceptualization of the Costs of Disease and Illness

Economic		Social
Direct	*Indirect*	
Prevention	Losses in output	Pain and suffering
Diagnosis	Lost time from work	Psychosocial deterioration
Treatment		Loss of body part
Hospitals, nursing homes		Impaired speech
Physician, nurses services		Disfigurement
Drugs		Disability
Medical research		Grief
Medical personnel training		Economic dependence
Facility construction		Social isolation
Public health education		Lost opportunities for promotion
		Relocation
		Changes in life plans
		Reduced self-esteem
		Resentment
		Mental disorders
		Sexual dysfunction
		Personality changes

Source: D. P. Rice and T. A. Hodgson, "Social and Economic Implications of Cancer in the United States," *Vital and Health Statistics* 3:20 (1981).

expenditures associated with prevention, diagnosis, and treatment. Indirect costs include such items as time lost from work and losses in output. Indirect costs can be valuated in economic terms, for example, by costing out the lost wages if a person has to stay home. Social costs are more difficult to assess in economic terms. Social costs include pain and suffering, psychosocial deterioration, loss of a body part, impaired speech, reduced self-esteem, and personality changes. On occasion researchers have applied "shadow pricing" techniques to associate dollar value with social costs.[68] It is noteworthy, however, that social costs may extend beyond the sick person to include families, friends, coworkers, and caregivers. Because they are difficult to evaluate, social costs are often reported directly. For example, various psychometric scales may be used to measure self-esteem and social isolation, and the results summarized statistically.

At the conceptual level, I think we have done a reasonable job of sorting out the various economic and noneconomic consequences of disease and illness. As is apparent from the definitions offered previously, social costs can be used to summarize the sick person's *illness*, while both direct and indirect economic costs best characterize the patient's *disease*. Thus, both the economic and sociological conceptualizations of disease and illness are nicely congruent. The most significant problems to be resolved concern the empirical assessment of both economic and social costs. The ability to measure these costs is now quite impressive, but, as described below, the manner in which we have chosen to go about this is inherently deficient. We must begin to consider the merits of a life course perspective on health care costs and our empirical data analysis techniques must be modified to fit our conceptualization of the course of chronic disease.

Diseases are typically described as infectious or chronic. Both may eventually result in death, and under such circumstances can be considered terminal. Historically infectious diseases have been the leading cause of death in the United States. Today this has changed largely because of preventive measures, including mass immunization, disease screening, and widespread changes in life-style. Prevention has extended the lives of most people and, as a result, chronic diseases and disorders, rather than those that are infectious, constitute the major causes of death. Despite our best efforts to the contrary, as people age they become increasingly susceptible to disease and more likely to become disabled.[69] While there are likely to be significant developments in the treatment of chronic disabling disease, it is improbable that such diseases will be successfully eradicated. Death will continue to be an inevitable event and will be the result of disease, accident, suicide, or homicide, as shown in Table 5.10. Nonetheless, postponement of death remains perhaps the most significant and established goal of medicine.

The distinction we maintain between infectious (often short-term) and chronic (long-term) disease has influenced the manner in which we conceptualize health care costs. Even in instances where chronic disease is the target of investigation, costs are almost always arrayed according to episodes of illness. In other words, when hospitalization is required, there is a tendency to treat the hospital *discharge* not the *patient* as the primary unit of analysis.[70] Because of this, the assessment of expenditures is focused on a relatively short-term experience—an initial encounter with little follow-up care. This episodic conceptualization of costs, as I will refer to it, is useful, but only for the examination of infectious diseases or acute disorders. Chronic disease, alternatively, requires a much broader long-term approach. In the treatment of chronic diseases and disorders, health care is required for an extended period of time. In

TABLE 5.10
Ten Leading Causes of Death in the United States, 1985

Rank	Cause of Death	Deaths	Percent of Total
1	Diseases of heart	775,890	37.2
2	Malignant neoplasms[a]	457,670	22.0
3	Cerebrovascular diseases	152,710	7.3
4	Accidents and adverse effects	92,070	4.4
5	Chronic obstructive pulmonary diseases, allied conditions	74,420	3.6
6	Pneumonia, influenza	66,630	3.2
7	Diabetes mellitus	38,620	1.9
8	Suicide	28,620	1.4
9	Chronic liver disease, cirrhosis	26,770	1.3
10	Atherosclerosis	23,580	1.1

Note: Total deaths equal 2.084 million. The ten leading causes of death account for 82.3 percent of all deaths. [a] Includes neoplasms of lymphotic and hematopoietic tissues.

Source: National Center for Health Statistics, "Annual Summary of Births, Marriages, Divorces, and Deaths: United States, 1985," *Monthly Vital Statistics Report* 34 (1986):21–22.

fact, barring a medical miracle that resolves the chronicity, the patient will require care for the remainder of his or her life. To understand the costs of such diseases, therefore, we must attempt to accumulate the necessary data longitudinally.

Perhaps we persistently ignore the long-term nature of chronic illness because of the analytic expediency of conceptualizing chronic disease costs as infectious, acute care costs. This, of course, is a valid approach provided that our interest is narrowly defined as a treatment episode in the trajectory of a chronic disease. Often, however, the goal of such analyses is to extrapolate beyond the episode of illness in an effort to gain a greater understanding of the health care costs associated with the treatment of chronic disease over the long term. In short, due to constraints imposed by available data, investigators opt to "make-do" with nonideal data in the hope that they are at least able to draw some valuable inferences. This has been true to some extent as we have become sensitive to the issues that surround "high-cost" illness.

Unfortunately, we have probably learned all we can from an episodic approach to disease costs. It is now time to access suitable data, or to collect the necessary data longitudinally, to understand the total financial implications of chronic disabling disease. Indeed, greater emphasis must be placed on longitudinal data than on episodic, cross-sectional data. We must develop a life-cycle perspective on health care costs, which includes both high-cost illness episodes requiring short-term treatment as well as maintenance therapy or continuing care required by patients over their lifetimes. Although the majority of people have an extended period in their lives when relatively little medical care is required, they eventually succumb to chronic disease or disability, unless accidental death intervenes. Both chronicity and disability impact significantly upon health care and related costs—chronic illness leads to increased health care expenditures directly and disability to long-term care needs.

This problem has been recognized by others. Perhaps the most exemplary work along these lines is that of Zook et al. In a rather detailed analysis of the records of patients undergoing treatment in "six contrasting hospital populations" in Massachusetts, Zook et al. " . . . examined the fiscal and clinical nature of repeated hospitalization for the same disease." The records for each patient in the study were linked across earlier hospitalizations to provide a longitudinal profile of repeated admissions. While their study had distinct advantages over previous studies, Zook et al. recognized the inherent shortcomings of their approach—multiple (different) illnesses were not studied and data collection was limited to the illness causing the current (index) admission.[71] They did, however, link data from other hospitals where a specific patient was treated if the hospital was in the study sample.

More recently, in a somewhat more limited analysis already commented upon, Berki et al. have attempted to compile data on twenty-seven acute care facilities in Maryland for calendar years 1979, 1980, and 1981.[72] These hospitals maintained "unit records" that allowed data to be linked both across disease episodes and hospitals. Even these data are limited, however, because they did not include information on physician charges for hospital stays and it was impossible to track hospital expenditures patients may have incurred at hospitals not included in the study sample.

To be sure, there are few studies of the type which will probably become increasingly important as we confront the difficult economic problems associated with the provision of health care. We must get away from narrowly conceived episodic approaches to health care costs; also we must realize the value of examining the costs of *maintaining* a life, not just the costs of *saving* a life. While we now face the moral and ethical dilemmas associated with saving lives, poignantly exemplified by organ transplantation, I am uncertain when we begin to ask whether it is worthwhile to maintain an individual's life in instances where the drama of death is less intense. Organ transplantation immediately places us amidst the life and death crucible as it were. Other sick persons whose ultimate demise is certain but lingering, are more difficult to reconcile on moral and ethical grounds. Of course the issue is that of discontinuing or withholding treatment. Why treat if we know we will be unsuccessful? Why treat if death is imminent? Why treat if we only prolong the death experience of a desperately ill patient?

Unfortunately, while the research my colleagues and I have pursued on transplantation has addressed virtually every thorny issue, the work remains incomplete. Our analysis of costs has been largely episodic, although we are well aware that the future of many transplant recipients is both uncertain and highly variable. We do know that transplantation and its accompanying treatment can give rise to a variety of serious medical complications. What we see, however, is the willingness on behalf of patients to "go for it." As many patients reflect on their experience, they do not hesitate to note that the alternative—death—is not attractive. If it were, why gamble with the transplant? Most patients recognize the risks associated with transplantation and envision themselves as risk takers. Most have gained some satisfaction out of living on the brink of disaster. The fear of death has been reconciled with the experience of dying. This perhaps accounts for many patients' relative insensitivity about economic costs while they are in an all-out pursuit to minimize the social costs associated with their illness.

The Concept of Risk in Relationship to Preventive Health Care

It is fashionable today to argue that preventive medicine represents a more reasonable allocation of health care resources than do costly technologies such as organ transplants, particularly heart and liver transplants.[73] This is not surprising, given present-day cost-containment objectives. However, the preventive health care argument amounts to little more than "wishing" away a deep-seated problem within the health care delivery system. What must be considered is that we have an aging population that at some point will encounter chronic or catastrophic disease which, in turn, can result in disability and excessive medical care expenditures. In short, all people will die, many with a chronic disabling disease that is costly to treat. To suggest that all disease and its attendant problems can be avoided indefinitely, as the preventionists seem to imply, represents a failure to come to grips with real world phenomena.

The preventionist ideology is also subject to criticism on the ground that preventive health care strategies can be as cost-ineffective as major catastrophic health care interventions. Central to the goal of prevention is the concept of risk reduction. The goal of preventive measures is to reduce the likely occurrence of ill health. The goal is laudable but the methods available to achieve it deceiving. For example, where should the line be drawn in determining precisely how far to go in attempting to minimize an untoward health effect? Do we isolate people from their environment to achieve the greatest period of life prolongation? Do we require that people behave in the most risk-aversive manner possible? Table 5.11 provides information on the estimated risk of death from various human-caused and natural accidents. To prevent deaths, do we discourage automobile and air travel? Do we make private swimming pools illegal? Do we require people to stay indoors during electrical storms? Where to draw the line to achieve health care objectives presents both a medical and a social dilemma. In short, the preventionists must demonstrate empirically that their goal can be achieved cost-effectively, and that it is possible to determine which efforts are most laudable.

In a detailed analysis of preventive health care measures, Russell argues that, "While prevention has great potential, it is neither riskless nor costless." Russell concluded the following:

> The evidence shows that, even after allowing for savings in treatment, prevention usually adds to medical expenditures, contrary to the popular view that it reduces them. . . . Prevention is not the solution to the problem of rising medical expenditures. These results show that prevention cannot be assumed to be a better choice than cure in every case. Individual measures must be evaluated on their own merits. To date few studies have been done that attempt direct comparisons between prevention and acute care.[74]

Certainly good health is valued and one cannot argue that prevention is an unworthy cause. However, prevention must be ". . . balanced against

TABLE 5.11
Estimated Risk of Death to an Individual from Various Human-Caused and Natural Accidents

Automobile accident	1 in 4,000
Drowning	1 in 30,000
Air travel	1 in 100,000
Lightning	1 in 2 million
Nuclear reaction accident	1 in 5 billion

Source: C. D. Klaassen, "Principles of Toxicology," in C. D. Klaassen, M. O. Amdur, J. Doull, eds., *Toxicology: The Basic Science of Poisons* (New York: MacMillan Publishing Co., 1986), pp. 11–32.

the costs to decide whether a particular measure is a good investment."[75]

Another popular misconception associated with prevention is the magnification of effect. This refers to the tendency to generalize the benefits of prevention beyond their appropriate boundaries. For example, we may successfully prevent one person from contracting cancer, but he or she may die of heart disease or in an automobile accident. Whereas the costs associated with the care of a cancer patient have been averted, the costs associated with other health care problems are not. Nearly 50 percent of all Americans die in hospitals, many requiring specialized or intensive care until death. Prevention will not avert this fact of life. In fact, life prolongation, even that attributable to preventive health initiatives, is a two-edged sword. Prolonging life simply increases the probability that expensive life-saving interventions may be required, even when such efforts are futile. It is not clear that the prolongation of life should necessarily be the foremost goal of medical care.

The changing age composition of the U.S. population assures us of complicated health problems in the future.[76] As people age, chronic disease and disability become more prevalent. We will essentially see a change in the character of disease from which old people succumb. For example, vaccines for pneumonia and influenza assure us that people will increasingly die of conditions for which the use of highly technological treatment will be indicated. The major moral dilemmas we will eventually face will be deciding what types of treatment should be applied to which types of patients. Should the eighty-five-year-old patient with renal failure be placed on maintenance dialysis? Should antibiotic treatment be provided to a terminally ill patient who has contracted pneumonia? These are not easy questions to answer, but they do represent the failures of our success in medicine.

Valuing Life

Placing a dollar value on human life has always been a matter of debate and the decision is often made to avoid rather than confront the controversies engendered by such an exercise.[77] Some would argue that since human life is priceless, no economic or clinical constraints should be imposed in pursuit of saving lives. Nevertheless, we both implicitly and explicitly discriminate in the medical treatment of individuals who are believed to be somewhat dispensable. For example, we do not offer the same type, level, and extent of health care to the poor and the elderly as are enjoyed and paid for by the more wealthy among us. Many hospitals catering to the medically indigent do not offer the same quality of services as hospitals whose caseloads are composed primarily of the privately insured. Perhaps this is simply another method by which we maintain social class distinctions within our society and extend our Darwinistic tendencies to medicine.

In the literature, several approaches have been presented to carry out the unattractive exercise of differentially valuing human lives. Culyer has identified the following: (1) the social decision approach, (2) the human capital approach, and (3) the risk-avoidance approach.[78]

The first approach looks at the resources a society has committed to saving a life. For example, one would attempt to determine the amount of money committed to traffic and highway safety projects and their relationship to deaths averted.

The human capital approach takes the social decision approach several steps further by attempting to impute a value to output lost due to ill health and death.[79] This approach imputes the discounted present value of expected future earnings, allowing for expected unemployment, average age of "victims," and other relevant factors. There is little question that this "social worth" approach to valuing lives undervalues the lives of children, homemakers, and retired persons since it adopts the view that people are "worth" only what they "contribute" to national output.

The third approach—the risk-avoidance approach—seeks to establish the maximum amount an individual would pay to effect a reduction in the probability of death. While conceptually more attractive than the human capital approach, the risk avoidance approach is somewhat difficult to apply directly.

By default, I think that today we are forced to use the social decision approach to get a handle on the value of human life. While imperfect, it does give us a starting point. I would argue further that the going rate, as it were, for a human life is approximately $25,000 per life-year. This estimate is based on our experience with the End-Stage Renal Disease program. I am sure, however, that we can find many exceptions—cases where a public or private payer incurs costs exceeding $25,000 per year per patient, and, of course, there are many, many cases where the amount is considerably less.

It seems to me that if we are to formulate health care coverage policies that are consistent, we must attempt to draw a threshold cost per year of life saved to decide how we will spend our health care dollar. This, of course, is the penultimate goal of cost-effectiveness analysis, and is the approximate approach we took to determine the clinical status of heart transplantation. What we were able to show was that heart transplantation was equally if not more cost-effective than other approaches covered by private and public insurers to treat patients with terminal illness. If we choose not to cover heart transplants, we must reconsider coverage of certain other medical interventions and treatments such as renal dialysis, the severely burned, etc.[80]

This approach, which constitutes a rather crude method of valuing lives, is useful. We may disagree with where the line should be drawn, but we can hardly disagree with the procedures to be followed. It seems to me that we must formulate health care policies that are fair, equitable, publicly accountable, and publicly defensible. To do otherwise will only assure us of the demise of our current health care delivery system. As long as we adhere to basic democratic principles, they will continue to provide the basic framework within which health care decisions will be made. National health insurance has not been rejected because its goal is objectionable but because of the basic philosophical and political beliefs which serve as its underpinnings.

Increasingly I find myself perplexed with the state of disarray that seems to characterize every aspect of our health care delivery system.[81] It seems that a certain measure of medical and social Darwinism is being infused into the system. While cost-effectiveness analysis is a reasonable tool to help us make difficult decisions, this is an inherently discriminatory approach—older, sicker patients will always be at a disadvantage.[82] If we adhere to the basic premise of the technique, a younger person would always be selected over an older person and a healthy person over a sicker one. In some respects, this constitutes a type of medical Darwinism and, as our resources become increasingly constrained, we will become even more Darwinistic in our approach to treating people.

Coincidentally, I am beginning to see a reemergence of social Darwinism—also embedded in the basic principles of cost-effectiveness analysis.[83] As described above, disease has both economic and social costs. While every effort is being made to contain economic costs (direct and indirect), we are also becoming less tolerant of social costs, particularly if patients require income support on behalf of public programs, such as those intended for the disabled. In this regard, the major findings of the National Kidney Dialysis and Kidney Transplantation Study are relevant.

- Nearly two-thirds of the ESRD patient population is receiving income support either through Social Security or the Supplemental Security Income program.
- Despite the foregoing benefits, nearly one-third of ESRD patients are living in households with incomes below the poverty line.
- Although income transfers to households through federal programs appear to raise many households above the poverty line, the major-

> ity of ESRD patients in poor families receive benefits that are insufficient to place them above the poverty threshold.

As these results suggest, treatment costs are only one aspect of the cost of illness—income support constitutes another aspect with sizable economic consequences. Is it surprising, therefore, that the present administration is considering reducing the number of persons who qualify for disability benefits? The extent to which this has untoward consequences for persons who are in bona fide need of assistance will be indicative of the degree to which social Darwinism has emerged as philosophically and politically acceptable.

While the foregoing discussion may appear radical, I assure you that it is not. Also, it is my contention that what is going on today is merely an accentuation of what has gone on in the past. Human lives are not of equal worth in our society. We can only more or less downplay the magnitude and significance of these differences. Sociologically speaking, class, status, and power do make a difference in the type of medical care received. Why, for example, was the president recently attended by a team of physicians brought in from the Mayo Clinic? How many people within our society have an equal level of choice?

We cannot, it seems to me, assure that everyone in our society receives an equal level of care, nor can I think of any society that is capable of making this guarantee. We can only try to minimize the differences, and in so doing, be cognizant of the fact that unavoidably we differentially value life. Sociologically, there is at least one school of thought—structural functionalism—that would argue that not only is this true, but it is entirely acceptable.

Conclusion

Organ transplantation typifies the broad range of problems that are associated with the treatment of catastrophic disease. It also demonstrates the public policy conflicts that arise when we consider the goals of medicine and our inability to economically satisfy these goals. For example, because of concerns about excessive program expenditures, should we vigorously attempt to increase the supply of donor organs? Would it not be better to curtail the supply of donor organs through preventive health care efforts? Alternatively, should we curtail efforts to prevent suicide since each potential victim could save the lives of several people? Clearly, we can identify a perverse set of objectives, not all of which we may be willing to endorse in the name of maximally saving lives. If, however, we are unwilling to make the necessary economic commitment to saving lives, it seems unfair to become too aggressive in our organ donation campaigns.

Cost-effectiveness analysis is valuable, but the implications of the widescale application of this approach to critical health care decisions indicate the need for caution. I say this, but recognize at the same time that this approach and its associated assumptions have completely infused our health care decision-making process. We are attracted to pragmatism despite our philosophical ambivalence. Discrimination is not a favorite goal of democracy.

Prevention of catastrophic maladies seems a laudable although overly simplistic approach. Human lives are spared at considerable expense, and prevention carries its cost. Preventive measures can be deployed as cost-ineffectively as any aggressive halfway technology.[84] In virtually every instance of catastrophic disease I am sure that medical professionals would prefer that they not have the problem to treat. However, in the absence of the problem, would the physician and staff be employed? Preventive medicine is not a prestigious or even a desirable specialty in medicine. Preventive dentistry has had a negative impact on the dental profession, and preventive medicine could have similar consequences for the practice of medicine.

Unlike many approaches to the treatment of catastrophic disease, organ transplantation has two associated resource allocation problems. First is the obvious issue of donor organ availability, a chronic problem. Second are problems associated with cost. If program expenditures were to increase to a level commensurate with an increase in the supply of donor organs, would we be willing to underwrite the costs? I am uncertain of this primarily because of the overall emphasis on cost containment. Increasingly, insurers are assessing larger beneficiary deductibles and copayments. Is it not likely that transplantation would serve to underscore these efforts?

How will we resolve, or at least address, the problem of differentially valuing life? Rising medical costs as well as income support expenditures are likely to spur greater interest in the unattractive exercise of placing a dollar value on human life. Again, transplants merely make such decisions a bit more poignant. As we gradually come to grips with the prevalence of the uninsured and the underinsured segment of our population as well as the long-term care needs of the elderly, I doubt that the topic of valuing lives will be avoided.

Certainly, an excessive amount of attention has focused on organ transplantation. Some would argue an unjustifiable amount. This may be true, but what we stand to gain from the viewpoint of public health policy is considerable. It is important that we take stock of what we have learned and apply it to other areas where our health care policies need development and/or elaboration.

Notes

1. R. W. Evans, "Heart Transplants and Priorities," *Lancet* 1 (1984):852–853; R. W. Evans, "Heart Transplants," *Issues in Science and Technology* 2 (1986):15, 123; and W. Casscells, "Heart Transplantation: Recent Policy Developments," *New England Journal of Medicine* 315 (1986):1365–1368.

2. Casscells, "Heart Transplantation."

3. L. B. Russell, *Is Prevention Better than Cure?* (Washington, D.C.: The Brookings Institution, 1986).

4. R. W. Evans, "The Heart Transplant Dilemma," *Issues in Science and Technology* 2 (1986):91–101.

5. R. W. Evans, C. R. Blagg, and F. A. Bryan, Jr., "Implications for Health Care Policy: A Social and Demographic Profile of Hemodialysis Patients in the United States," *Journal of the American Medical Association* 245 (1981):487–491; and R. A. Rettig, *Implementing the End-Stage Renal Disease Program of Medicare* (Santa Monica, Ca.: The Rand Corporation, 1980).

6. G. Calabresi and P. Bobbitt, *Tragic Choices* (New York: Norton and Co., 1978); and J. F. Childress, *Who Should Decide? Paternalism in Health Care* (New York: Oxford University Press, 1982).

7. L. E. Goodman and M. J. Goodman, "Prevention—How Misuse of a Concept Undercuts its Worth," *Hastings Center Report* 16 (1986):26–38.

8. P. W. Eggers, "Impact of Transplantation on the Medicare ESRD Program," in press.

9. D. R. Waldo, K. R. Levit, and H. Lazenby, "National Health Care Expenditures, 1985," *Health Care Financing Review* 8 (1986):1–21.

10. Waldo et al., "National Health Care Expenditures, 1985."

11. R. W. Evans, "Health Care Technology and the Inevitability of Resource Allocation and Rationing Decisions," Parts 1 and 2, *Journal of the American Medical Association* 249 (1983):2047–2053, 2208–2219.

12. R. W. Evans et al., *The National Heart Transplantation Study: Final Report, Volumes 1-5* (Seattle: Battelle Human Affairs Research Centers, 1984); R. W. Evans et al., *The Treatment of End-Stage Renal Disease in the U.S.: Selected Findings from the National Kidney Dialysis and Kidney Transplantation Study* (Baltimore: Health Care Financing Administration, in press); and National Task Force on Organ Transplantation, *Final Report* (Rockville, Md.: Health Resources and Services Administration, 1986).

13. Evans et al., "Implications for Health Care Policy"; R. W. Evans et al., "The Need for and Supply of Donor Hearts for Transplantation," *Heart Transplantation* 4 (1984):57–62; R. W. Evans et al., "Donor Availability as the Primary Determinant of the Future of Heart Transplantation," *Journal of the American Medical Association* 255 (1986):1892–1898; and R. W. Evans, "Coverage and Reimbursement for Heart Transplantation," *International Journal of Technology Assessment in Health Care* 2 (1986):425–449.

14. R. W. Evans, "Cost Effectiveness Analysis of Transplantation," *Surgical Clinics of North America* 66 (1986):603–616; and R. W. Evans, "The Socioeconomics of Organ Transplantation," *Transplantation Proceedings* 17 (Suppl) (1985):129–136.

15. Evans et al., "Need for and Supply of Donor Hearts"; Evans et al., "Donor Availability"; and National Center for Health Statistics, "Annual Summary of Births, Marriages, Divorces, and Deaths: United States, 1985," *Monthly Vital Statistics Report* 34 (1986):1–28.

16. Evans et al., "National Heart Transplantation Study."

17. K. Merriken and T. D. Overcast, "Patient Selection for Heart Transplantation: When is a Discriminating Choice Discrimination?" *Journal of Health Politics, Policy and Law* 10 (1985):7–32.

18. Evans et al., "Need for and Supply of Donor Hearts"; Evans et al., "Donor Availability"; T. D. Overcast et al., "Problems in the Identification of Potential Organ Donors," *Journal of the American Medical Association* 251 (1984):1559–1562; and D. L. Manninen and R. W. Evans, "Public Attitudes and Behavior Regarding Organ Donation," *Journal of the American Medical Association* 253 (1985):3111–3115.

19. National Task Force, *Final Report.*

20. Evans et al., "Donor Availability."

21. N. L. Ascher and R. W. Evans, "Designation of Liver Transplant Centers in the United States," *Transplant Proceedings* 19 (1987):2405.

22. National Task Force, *Final Report.*

23. T. A. H. English et al., "Selection and Procurement of Hearts for Transplantation," *British Medical Journal* 288 (1984):1889–1891; and R. W. Emery et al., "The Cardiac Donor: A Six-Year Experience," *Annals of Thoracic Surgery* 41 (1986):356–362.

24. R. W. Evans, *The Proliferation of Cardiac Transplant Facilities: Results of a Survey of Hospitals with Open-Heart Surgery Facilities* (Seattle, Wa.: Battelle Human Affairs Research Centers, 1985).

25. Evans et al., "Donor Availability."

26. J. G. Copeland et al., "The Total Artificial Heart as a Bridge-to Transplant," *Journal of the American Medical Association* 256 (1986):2991–2995; L. D. Joyce et al., "Summary of the World Experience with Clinical Use of Total Artificial Hearts as Heart Support Devices," *Journal of Heart Transplantation* 5 (1986):229–235; M. M. Levinson et al., "Three Recent Cases of the Total Artificial Heart Before Transplantation," *Journal of Heart Transplantation* 5 (1986):215--228; B. P. Griffith et al., "Use of the Total Artificial Heart as an Interim Device: Initial Experience in Pittsburgh with Four Patients," *Journal of Heart Transplantation* 5 (1986):210–214; L. D. Joyce et al., "Use of the Mini Jarvik-7 Total Artificial Heart as a Bridge to Transplantation," *Journal of Heart Transplantation* 5 (1986):203–209; J. A. Magovern et al., "Bridge to Heart Transplantation: The Penn State Experience," *Journal of Heart Transplantation* 5 (1986):196–202; H. M. Cole, "Four Years of Replacing Ailing Hearts: Surgeons Assess Data, Questions Remain," *Journal of the American Medical Association* 256 (1986):2921–2925, 2929–2930; and A. S. Relman, "Artificial Hearts–Permanent and Temporary," *New England Journal of Medicine* 315 (1986):1029.

27. D. P. Lubeck and J. P. Bunker, *The Artificial Heart: Costs, Risks, and Benefits (Case Study/9)* (Washington, D.C.: Office of Technology Assessment, 1982).

28. The Working Group on Mechanical Circulatory Support of the National Heart, Lung, and Blood Institute, *Artificial Heart and Assist Devices: Directions, Needs, Costs, Societal and Ethical Issues* (Bethesda, Md.: National Heart, Lung and Blood Institute, 1985).

29. R. S. Mecklenburg et al., "Long-term Metabolic Control with Insulin Pump Therapy: Report of Experience with 127 Patients," *New England Journal of Medicine* 313 (1985):465–468; D. S. Schade and R. P. Eaton, "Insulin Delivery: How, When, and Where," *New England Journal of Medicine* 312 (1985):1120–1121; S. J. Brink and C. Stewart, "Insulin Pump Treatment in Insulin-Dependent Diabetes Mellitus," *Journal of the American Medical Association* 255 (1986):617–621; D. R. Coustan et al., "A Randomized Clinical Trial of the Insulin Pump Versus Intensive Conventional Therapy in Diabetic Pregnancies," *Journal of the American Medical Association* 255 (1986):631–636; and F. K. Thorp, "Insulin Pump Therapy Reconsidered," *Journal of the American Medical Association* 255 (1986):645–647.

30. K. Reemtsma et al., "Renal Heterotransplantation in Man," *Annals of Surgery* 160 (1964):384–410; T. E. Starzl et al., "Renal Heterotransplantation from Baboon to Man: Experience with 6 Cases," *Transplantation* 2 (1964):752–776; J. D. Hardy et al., "Heart Transplantation in Man," *Journal of the American Medical Association* 188 (1964):114–122; L. L. Bailey et al., "Orthotopic Cardiac Transplantation in Cyclosporine-Treated Neonate," *Transplant Proceedings* 15 (1983):2956–2959; L. L. Bailey et al., "Baboon-to-Human Cardiac Xenotransplantation in a Neonate," *Journal of the American Medical Association* 254 (1985):3321–3329; L. L. Bailey et al., "Host Maturation Afer Orthotopic Cardiac Transplantation During Neonatal Life," *Heart Transplantation* 3 (1984):265–267; and J. G. Losman, "Heart Xenotransplantation in a Newborn," *Journal of Heart Transplantation 4 (1984):10–11.*

31. Losman, "Heart Xenotransplantation."

32. J. M. Prottas, "Obtaining Replacements: The Organizational Framework of Organ Procurement," *Journal of Health Politics, Policy and Law* 8 (1983):235–250; J. M. Prottas, "Encouraging Altrusion: Public Attitudes and the Marketing of Organ Donation," *Milbank Memorial Fund Quarterly/Health and Society* 61 (1983):278–306; J. M. Prottas, "Organ Procurement in Europe and the United States," *Milbank Memorial Fund Quarterly/Health and Society* 63 (1985):94–126; J. M. Prottas, "The Structure and Effectiveness of the U.S. Organ Procurement System," *Inquiry* 22 (1986):365–376.

33. A. L. Caplan, "Ethical and Policy issues in the Procurement of Cadaver Organs for Transplantation," *New England Journal of Medicine* 311 (1984):981–983; and T. E. Starzl, "Implied Consent for Cadaveric Organ Donation," *Journal of the American Medical Association* 251 (1984):1592.

34. Evans et al., "Donor Availability."

35. Anonymous, "Wearing Seat Belts Reduces Car Casualties," *Lancet* 2 (1983):1377; Notes and News, "Seat Belts Reduce Serious Injury," *Lancet* 1 (1984):975; and A. F. Williams and A. K. Lund, "Seat Belt Laws and Occupant Crash Protection in the United States," *American Journal of Public Health* 76 (1986):1438–1442.

36. A. F. Williams and J. K. Wells, "The Tennessee Child Restraint Law in its

Third Year," *American Journal of Public Health* 71 (1981):163–165; M. D. Decker et al., "The Use and Efficacy of Child Restraint Devices," *Journal of the American Medical Association* 252 (1984):2571–2575; R. S. Sanders and B. B. Dan, "Bless the Seats and the Children: The Physician and the Legislative Process," *Journal of the American Medical Association* 252 (1984):2613–2614; D. Guerin and D. P. MacKinnon, "An Assessment of the California Child Passenger Restraint Requirement," *American Journal of Public Health* 75 (1985):142–144; P. F. Agran and P. F. Wehrle, "Injury Reduction by Mandatory Child Passenger Safety Laws," *American Journal of Public Health* 75 (1985):128–129; and A. K. Fuller, A. E. Fuller, and L. E. Yates, "The Use of Child Restraint Devices in Vehicles," *Journal of the American Medical Association* 255 (1986):614.

37. Evans, "Cost Effectiveness Analysis of Transplantation"; and Evans, "Socioeconomics of Organ Transplantation."

38. S. A. Finkler, "The Distinction Between Costs and Charges," *Annals of Internal Medicine* 96 (1982):102–109.

39. Evans et al., "National Heart Transplantation Study."

40. T. F. O'Donnell et al., "The Economic Impact of Acute Variceal Bleeding: Cost Effectiveness Implications for Medical and Surgical Therapy," *Surgery* 88 (1980):693–701.

41. Evans et al., "National Heart Transplantation Study."

42. J. Lubitz and R. Prihoda., "The Use and Costs of Medicare Services in the Last Two Years of Life," *Health Care Financing Review* 5 (1984):117–131.

43. Lubitz and Prihoda, "Use and Costs of Medicare."

44. N. McCall, "Utilization and Costs of Medicare Services by Beneficiaries in their Last Year of Life," *Medical Care* 22 (1984):329–342; A. A. Scitovsky, "'The High Cost of Dying:' What Do the the Data Show?" *Milbank Memorial Fund Quarterly/Health and Society* 62 (1984):591–608; W. D. Spector and V. Mor, "Utilization and Charges for Terminal Cancer Patients in Rhode Island," *Inquiry* 21 (1984):328–337; S. H. Long et al., "Medical Expenditures of Terminal Cancer Patients During the Last Year of Life," *Inquiry* 21 (1984):315–327; B. S. Bloom, R. S. Knorr, and A. E. Evans, "The Epidemiology of Disease Expenses: The Cost of Caring for Children with Cancer," *Journal of the American Medical Association* 253 (1985):2393–2397; and A. A. Scitovsky and A. M. Capron, "Medical Care at the End of Life: The Interaction of Economics and Ethics," in L. Breslow, ed., *Annual Review of Public Health,* 1986 (Palo Alto, Ca.: Annual Reviews, Inc., 1986).

45. Evans et al., *Treatment of End-Stage Renal Disease.*

46. Eggers, "Impact of Transplantation."

47. Eggers, "Impact of Transplantation."

48. W. L. Roper, "Medicare Program Criteria for Medicare Coverage of Heart Transplants," *Federal Register* 51 (17 October 1986):37164--37170.

49. Health Insurance Association of America, *Organ Transplants and Their Implications for the Health Insurance Industry* (Washington, D.C.: HIAA, 1985); D. L. Kastiel, "Insurers Want Controls on Transplant Costs," *Business Insurance,* 4 November 1985; and Blue Cross-Blue Shield, *Technology Evaluation and Coverage. Criteria for Evaluating Institutions for Liver and Heart Transplants* (Chicago: Health Benefits Management Division, Blue Cross-Blue Shield, 1985).

50. National Task Force, *Final Report.*

51. Evans et al., "National Heart Transplantation Study"; and Evans et al., *Treatment of End-Stage Renal Disease.*

52. National Task Force, *Final Report.*

53. R. W. Evans et al., "The Quality of Life of End-Stage Renal Disease Patients," *New England Journal of Medicine* 312 (1985):553–559; R. W. Evans et al., "The Quality of Life of Kidney and Heart Transplant Recipients," *Transplantation Proceedings* 17 (1985):1579–1582; N. D. Meister et al., "Returning to Work After Heart Transplantation," *Journal of Heart Transplantation* 5 (1986):154–161; and M. E. Lough, J. L. Miller, and P. Gamberg, "Self-Reported Change in Physical Symptoms from Cyclosporine-Based Therapy to Azathioprine-Based Therapy in Heart Transplant Recipients," *Journal of Heart Transplantation* 5 (1986):322–326.

54. Evans et al., "Quality of Life of End-Stage Renal Disease"; and Evans et al., "Quality of Life of Kidney and Heart Transplant Patients."

55. S. E. Berki et al., *High Cost Illness Among Hospitalized Patients. Final Report on Phase I of Contract No. 233-81-3021* (Springfield, Il.: National Technical Information Service; December 1983).

56. S. A. Schroeder, J. A. Showstack, and H. E. Roberts, "Frequency and Clinical Discretion of High-Cost Patients in 17 Acute-Care Hospitals," *New England Journal of Medicine* 300 (1979):1306–1309.

57. E. J. Kobrinski and A. L. Matteson, "Characteristics of High Cost Treatment in Acute Care Facilities," *Inquiry* 18 (1981):179–184.

58. H. Birnbaum, *A National Profile of Catastrophic Illness* (Hyattsville, Md.: National Center for Health Services Research, 1978); H. Birnbaum, *The Cost of Catastrophic Illness* (Lexington, Ma.: D.C. Heath and Co., 1978).

59. Congressional Budget Office, *Catastrophic Medical Expenses: Patterns in the Non-Elderly, Non-Poor Population* (Washington, D.C.: GPO, 1982).

60. Congressional Budget Office, *Catastrophic Health Insurance* (Washington, D.C.: GPO, 1977).

61. R. N. Forthofer, D. R. Lairson, and G. H. Glasson, "Catastrophic Health Insurance and HMOs," *Social Science in Medicine* 16 (1982):1775–1779.

62. Berki et al., "High Cost Illness."

63. Berki et al., "High Cost Illness."

64. Berki et al., "High Cost Illness."

65. National Task Force, *Final Report.*

66. Waldo et al., "Health Care Expenditures, 1985."

67. D. P. Rice, *Estimating the Cost of Illness* (Washington, D.C.: GPO, 1966); D. P. Rice, "Estimating the Cost of Illness," *American Journal of Public Health* 57 (1967):424–440; D. P. Rice and T. A. Hodgson, "Social and Economic Implications of Cancer in the United States," *Vital and Health Statistics* 3:20 (1981); and T. A. Hodgson and M. R. Meiners, "Cost-of-Illness Methodology: A Guide to Current Practices," *Milbank Memorial Fund Quarterly/Health and Society* 60 (1982):429–462.

68. C. C. Abt, "The Issue of Social Costs in Cost-Benefit Analysis of Surgery," in J. P. Bunker, B. A. Barnes, F. Mosteller, eds., *Costs, Risks, and Benefits of Surgery* (New York: Oxford University Press, 1977), pp. 40–55.

69. Evans, "Health Care Technology," parts 1 and 2.

70. Berki et al., "High Cost Illness;" and S. E. Berki et al., "High Volume and

Low Volume Users of Health Services, United States, 1980," *National Medical Care Utilization and Expenditure Survey* C:2 (1985).

71. C. J. Zook et al., "Repeated Hospitalizations for the Same Disease: A Multiplier of National Health Costs," *Milbank Memorial Fund Quarterly/Health and Society* 58 (1980):454–471.

72. Berki et al., "High Cost Illness."

73. Casscells, "Heart Transplantation."

74. Russell, "Is Prevention Better."

75. Russell, "Is Prevention Better."

76. Evans, "Health Care Technology," parts 1 and 2.

77. D. P. Rice, "The Economic Value of Human Life," *American Journal of Public Health* 57 (1967):1954–1966; W. I. Card and G. H. Mooney, "What is the Monetary Value of a Human Life," *British Medical Journal* 2 (1977):1627–1629; M. W. Jones-Lee, *The Value of Life: An Economic Analysis* (Chicago: University of Chicago Press, 1976); G. H. Mooney, *The Valuation of Human Life* (London: Macmillan Press, 1977); D. P. Rice and T. A. Hodgson, "The Value of Life Revisited," *American Journal of Public Health* 72 (1982):536–538; J. S. Landefeld and D. P. Seskin, "The Economic Value of Life: Linking Theory to Practice," *American Journal of Public Health* 72 (1982):555–566; M. S. Thompson, "Willingness to Pay and Accept Risks to Cure Chronic Disease," *American Journal of Public Health* 76 (1982):392–396; and N. S. Dorfman, "The Social Value of Saving a Life," in J. J. Muskin and D. Dunlop, eds., *Health: What is it Worth? Measures of Health Benefits* (New York: Pergamon Press, 1979), pp. 61–68.

78. A. J. Culyer, "Assessing Cost-Effectivenss," in H. D. Banta, ed., *Resources for Health: Technology Assessment for Policy Making* (New York: Praeger Publishers, 1982), pp. 107–120.

79. Rice, "Economic Value of Human Life"; and Rice and Hodgson, "Value of Life."

80. Evans, "Heart Transplantation Dilemma."

81. L. A. Coser, *Masters of Sociological Thought: Ideas in Historical and Social Context* (New York: Harcourt Brace Jovanovich, Inc., 1971), pp. 89–127; H. Spencer, *The Study of Sociology* (New York: Appleton, 1891); and H. Spencer, *The Principles of Sociology* (New York: Appleton, 1896).

82. J. Avorn, "Benefit and Cost Analysis in Geriatric Care: Turning Age Discrimination into Health Policy," *New England Journal of Medicine* 310 (1984):1294–1301; and P. Doubilet, M. C. Weinstein, and B. J. McNeil, "Use and Misuse of the Term 'Cost-Effective' in Medicine," *New England Journal of Medicine* 314 (1986):253–256.

83. Coser, *Masters of Thought;* and Spencer, *Principles of Sociology.*

84. Russell, "Is Prevention Better."

6

Aging Reconsidered: Emerging Research and Policy Issues

John W. Rowe and Robert H. Binstock

The phenomenon of population aging—or, as some have termed it, "the geriatric imperative"[1]—is becoming well recognized in contemporary society. We are becoming aware that 28 million Americans are now aged sixty-five and older, constituting about 12 percent of the population, that they account for one-third of annual health care expenditures in the United States, and that in the year 2000 this age group will number 35 million persons or about 13 percent of the nation's population.[2]

Less widely understood, however, is the fact that America's elderly population is continually changing in ways that have significant implications not only for the provision of health care but also for other activities and sectors in society.[3] We must recognize that "the aging" are a "moving target" in several important respects. This chapter considers several disparate emerging research and policy issues that are influenced by the rapidly changing nature of aging in America.

Aging in America: A Moving Target

The Changing Age Structure of the Older Population

The age distribution *within* the population aged sixty-five and older is changing markedly and will continue to do so. The tidal wave of elderly in the United States contains a second wave. The elderly themselves are growing older. Although persons aged eighty-five and over constituted only 8.8 percent of the American older population in 1980, in the year 2000 they will comprise 14 percent of the group. Similarly, in 1980 persons aged seventy-five and older constituted 39 percent of the older population, and by 2000 they will be 50 percent of it.[4]

For health care, the implications of this continuing shift toward an increasingly older "old-age" population are staggering. While 45 percent of all health care spending on persons aged sixty-five and older in the

United States is currently expended on hospitals,[5] this percentage is apt to rise dramatically since persons aged seventy-five to eighty-four use hospitals at a rate which is 69 percent higher than that of the sixty-five to seventy-four-year-old group,[6] a figure that rises to 113 percent for those older than eighty-five.

It is problematic, of course, to assume that treatment and prevention modalities, and especially the mechanisms of organizing, financing, and delivering health care will remain relatively static over the next ten to twenty years. But these comparisons among older age groups with respect to their hospital utilization rates should make it clear that no matter how the health care terrain evolves in the years ahead, the changing age structure within the older population will, in itself, have a substantial impact upon the nature and volume of the demand for acute care and the resources necessary to respond to it.

The changing age structure within the older population also portends a substantial increase in the demand for long-term care. Although "long-term care" is a conventional metaphor for health care and social supports for chronically ill and disabled *older* persons, it is a misleading metaphor. The fact is that there are more than twice as many severely disabled, noninstitutionalized adults (aged eighteen to sixty-four) in the United States than there are chronically ill and severely disabled persons aged sixty-five and older *both in and not in* institutions.[7] The changing distribution of age groups within the sixty-five and older category, however, suggests that the metaphor may become more accurate in the decades ahead.

The prevalence of many chronic disabling conditions rises exponentially after age seventy,[8] an effect reflected in an increased demand for care. In 1985, about 2 percent of persons aged sixty-five to seventy-four in the United States were in nursing homes; this compared with 7 percent of persons aged seventy-five to eighty-four, and 16 percent of persons aged eighty-five and older.[9] Consequently, the greater number of persons who soon will be in the older old-age categories underlies projections that the current nursing home population of 1.5 million persons will increase to 2.1 million by the year 2000, and reach 4.4 million some forty years later,[10] and will be accompanied by increases in the number of noninstitutionalized older persons who will be as severely disabled as those in nursing homes.[11]

It is possible, of course, that potential advances in preventing and treating urinary incontinence, osteoporosis, stroke, Alzheimer's Disease, and other conditions will delay the onset of chronic illness and disability to even older ages, which will reduce both the prevalence and duration of morbidity near the end of life. It is estimated, for instance, that modest reductions in the age-related rate of bone loss, delaying hip fracture to five years later than it currently occurs, would reduce the overall number of hip fractures by 50 percent! To date, however, there is no scientific evidence to support such an optimistic paradigm for a compression of morbidity.[12]

The Different Persons Who Constitute the Older Population

The cohort of older persons in this country is continuously changing because of its rapid turnover, due to birthdays and deaths. Estimates from Census data are that each day 5,200 Americans reach their sixty-fifth birthday and 3,600 persons who are sixty-five and older die.[13]

Over time, large new cohorts accumulate within the older population and others exit through death. These new cohorts of older persons will have lived through specific historical periods (i.e., immigration, the Great Depression, medical advances) at earlier stages in their lives than the cohorts they replace. Although not all members of a cohort will have been affected by earlier periods and events in the same fashion, the replacement of one cohort by another can result in substantial changes in the distribution of physical, social, and economic characteristics among older persons. Many of these changes have significant implications for the health status and health care of older persons.

One positive implication of such changes has been and will continue to be the improved oral health of the older population. New cohorts entering old age have lived through periods during which both personal oral hygiene and the quality and quantity of available dental care have undergone steady improvement. For instance, the percentage of Americans older than sixty-five who have no teeth has steadily declined from 55 percent in 1957, to 46 percent in 1973, and to 34 percent in 1980![14] Also, cohorts entering old age early in the next century will have been exposed at an early age to the public health intervention of fluoridated water systems, with the likely result of continued improvements in the dental health status of the older population.

Higher educational levels among newer cohorts may bode well for improvements in the extent to which they understand and comply with health care instructions and guidance, undertake better self-care, and seek medical assistance. The impact of the changing educational characteristics of older persons is such that in the two decades of 1970–1990 the median years of school completed by persons aged sixty-five years and older will have increased 37 percent.[15]

Some implications of cohort turnover, however, can be negative. For instance, coronary heart disease is currently more common among older men than women.[16] But increases in the prevalence of cigarette smoking among young and middle-aged females during the decades following World War II could lead to a marked change in the incidence of coronary disease among older women.

The Concept of Normality in Studies of Aging

Increasing interest in aging and the medical problems of older persons has fueled substantial growth in physiologic, psychologic, and sociologic research on aging. Investigators recognize the importance of separating pathologic from age-related changes. Thus, for physiologic studies careful guidelines are developed to exclude individuals whose profiles might not represent "normal" aging, and instead might be contaminated by changes related to specific disease processes.[17] In addition to focusing on community dwelling older persons with no history of illness or medication use, investigators now routinely obtain specific physiologic or biomedical measures in order to further assess their fitness for study and exclude individuals whose results lie beyond a reasonable statistical guideline, such as three standard deviations for their age group. Results for the remaining population are felt to represent "normal" aging, with more confidence regarding the age-specificity of the findings resting on longitudinal studies of age changes than cross-sectional comparisons of age differences which are sensitive to cohort effects.

Over the past thirty years numerous cross-sectional and longitudinal studies on carefully screened, well-characterized populations have demonstrated the major effects of age on clinically relevant variables, including hearing, vision, renal function, glucose tolerance, systolic blood pressure, bone density, pulmonary function, immune function, sympathetic nervous system activity, and a variety of cognitive and behavioral measures. Such nonpathologic aging effects are important to understand not only as reflections of the aging process, but also because they serve as a physiologic substrate for the influence of age on the presentation of disease, its response to treatment and the complications that ensue. However, this dichotomy of findings into disease-related versus "normal" aging has important limitations—it tends to neglect the substantial heterogeneity among older persons with regard to many physiologic and cognitive variables; it has tended to imply that the physiologic changes that occur in older individuals in the absence of disease are *harmless* and do not carry a significant risk. In short, the identification of certain physiologic changes as "normal" has tended to suggest that these changes are the natural state of affairs and thus cannot or should not be modified.

Successful and Usual Aging as Subtypes of Normal Aging

In the absence of disease, the physiologic changes that occur with "normal" aging are highly variable, are often associated with attributable risk for adverse health events, and are potentially modifiable. The intrinsic aging process may contribute less to decrements in aged populations than previously recognized. Factors such as personal habits, diet, exercise, nutrition, environmental exposures, and body composition may play more important roles than aging.

While many physiologic variables, including cardiovascular, immune, endocrine, renal, and pulmonary functions, show fairly substantial losses with advancing age, an important characteristic of these data sets regarding these functions is the substantial variability within them.[18] The variability often increases with age so that older people become less like each other rather than more like each other. In many data sets, one can easily find older persons with minimal or no physiologic loss compared to their younger counterparts, while the average change in the aged group is a substantial decrement from earlier results.

Rather than focusing purely on the differentiation of the effects of disease versus "normal" aging, gerontologic studies should recognize that the "normal" aging group includes two important subsets. The first comprises those individuals who demonstrate minimal age-associated losses in a given physiologic function (immune, bone density, carbohydrate tolerance, renal, cognitive, etc.). These individuals might be viewed as aging "successfully" with regard to the particular variable under study. Individuals who demonstrate "successful" aging in a constellation of physiologic functions, rather than in just one present minimal physiologic loss and robust physiologic function in advanced age—a pure aging syndrome. This successful aging group represents a small but potentially increasing portion of the overall "normal" aging population, the bulk of which is represented by the group that might be termed "usual" aging. For a given physiologic variable, the usual aging group has significant impairments when compared to their younger counterparts but do not qualify as diseased. The physiologic losses in the usual aging group display large interindividual differences and these individuals with the greatest "age effect" are at increased risk of developing a specific disease or disability.

The pathways of physiological or psychological change that individuals take with advancing age are influenced by intrinsic aging processes and a variety of extrinsic factors, including genetic and environmental influences, personal habits, diet, psychosocial factors, and diseases. We should also be aware that older persons who display "usual aging" for a given function may be able to improve their function and thus potentially reduce their risk of adverse outcomes. Thus, the focus of study is moving gradually from the evaluation of the emergence of diseases in an aging population to elucidation of the factors which regulate the transition of individuals from successful to usual states of aging and vice-versa.

This perspective of successful versus usual aging will be applied to a few physiologic and cognitive variables generally considered to decline significantly with normal aging.

Aging and Carbohydrate Metabolism

It has been known for over sixty years that advancing age is associated with progressive impairments in the capacity to metabolize a glucose challenge.[19] After excluding individuals with fasting hyperglycemia which is indicative of diabetes mellitus, and those treated with medications known to alter glucose tolerance and those expected to become diabetic, results of oral or intravenous glucose tolerance tests show a remarkable increase in the mean two-hour blood sugar level with advancing age. There also is a substantial increase in variability in successive age groups; many older individuals metabolize glucose as well as their average younger counterparts. Resistance to the effect of insulin on peripheral tissues appears to play a major role in the genesis of the glucose intolerance of aging. As with other insulin resistant states, the insulin resistance of aging is associated with progressive increases in postprandial insulin levels.[20]

The carbohydrate intolerance of aging may carry substantial risk. While several prospective epidemiologic studies suggest an increase in coronary heart disease risk with hyperglycemia in nondiabetics, an international collaborative group evaluating a total of fifteen such studies did not find consistent evidence for such an effect.[21] On the other hand, studies focusing on postprandial hyperinsulinemia, a cardinal feature of the insulin resistance of aging, have shown increases in insulin levels to be a significant contributor to the incidence of death from coronary heart disease.[22] In addition to these direct effects, increases in insulin level are associated with increases in triglyceride levels and decreases in high density lipoprotein-cholesterol levels—both of which are known risk factors for heart disease.[23]

Attempts have been made to determine which components of the age-associated alterations in carbohydrate intolerance are related to aging per se and which might be related to factors such as diet, exercise, medication, and body composition.

In Italian factory workers aged twenty-two to seventy-three, Zavaroni et al. evaluated the relative contributions of obesity, physical activity, family history of diabetes, and the use of diabetogenic drugs to the age-related increases in glucose and insulin levels after an oral glucose tolerance test.[24] The initial strong statistical correlation between age and both postprandial glucose and insulin levels became much weaker when the effects of exercise, diet, and drugs were taken into account, so that the correlation between glucose and age was limited to marginal statistical significance, and there was no longer an effect of age on insulin levels. Hollenbeck showed a direct significant relationship between physical fitness as reflected in maximal oxygen consumption and insulin-stimulated glucose metabolism in non-obese healthy older men.[25]

As pointed out by Reaven and Reaven these findings clearly suggest that much of the carbohydrate intolerance of aging may be related to factors other than normal biological aging per se, and also suggests that dietary or exercise modifications may substantially blunt the emergence of carbohydrate intolerance and insulin resistance with age.[26] This view is supported by previous studies demonstrating improvements in glucose tolerance in young adults and diabetics after exercise regimens as well as recent studies suggesting that exercise programs also improve the glucose intolerance and insulin resistance of aging.[27]

Aging and Osteoporosis

Aging is associated with a progressive decline in bone density in both males and females after maturity. Losses in bone density so severe as to result in fractures after minimal trauma define the "disease" osteoporosis which accounts for over 1 million fractures in the United States each year. Osteoporosis is of staggering importance in the elderly. By age sixty-five, one-third of women will have vertebral fractures and by age eighty-one, one-third of women and one-sixth of men will have suffered a hip fracture, often a catastrophic, if not terminal, event.[28]

While it has long been recognized that osteoporosis is a highly variable process with multiple possible causes, the normal aging process has generally been considered a major factor. In a review of current information regarding involutional osteoporosis, Riggs and Melton indicate that three separate components contribute to age-related bone loss.[29] The first component, the effect of intrinsic aging, represents a modest decline in bone mass with advancing age in both men and women and includes several identifiable physiologic processes. The second component, a more rapid decline in bone mass in women after middle age, is accountable to the effects of menopause. The third component, which is of potential major clinical importance, represents the net effect of "extrinsic" factors present to a variable degree in the population which contribute to the remarkable variance in bone density among the elderly. These preventable risk factors include cigarette smoking, heavy alcohol intake, and inadequate calcium intake.[30]

A number of studies suggest that bone loss is modifiable in advanced age by the institution of moderate exercise programs.[31] Thus, the emergence of osteoporosis, a common, crippling, and expensive disorder previously considered to represent the "normal" aging process, is variable and influenced by both aging and non-aging factors. The marked reductions in bone density associated with "usual" aging may be largely preventable or modifiable.

Aging and Cognitive Function

Parallel apparent age-related changes which on further study turn out to be not related to the intrinsic aging process and may be modifiable have been found in cognitive domains as well.[32] Schaie and his colleagues conducted a series of cross-sequential studies on successive cohorts of individuals across the adult age range which permit a comparison of cross-sectional and longitudinal data from the same study populations.[33] Subjects tested in 1963 demonstrated a decline in cognitive performance with advancing age. Interestingly, when the same subjects were retested seven years later, the age-related declines on tests of crystallized intelligence (such as verbal tests) and fluid intelligence, (such as inductive reasoning and spatial orientation) were significantly delayed until later ages. Clearly, such a difference reflects a well-known cohort effect where successive age cohorts demonstrate differences at the same chronological age due to changes not in the intrinsic aging process but in other factors that influence the variable being measured. Thus, while the results of the 1963 studies might have been viewed as characterizing the decline with aging in cognitive function much of that decline was clearly not a result of intrinsic aging but reflected sensitive differences between the younger and older cohorts. These differences clearly might be in educational level or health or nutritional factors that may have influenced the capacity to maintain neuropsychological integrity until later in age.

A demonstration of the important influence of education in determining the level of "usual" versus "successful" aging can be seen in Green's comparison of scores on the Wechsler Adult Intelligence Scale between a stratified random population sample in which there was a marked decline with age in educational level and an educationally balanced sample.[34] The stratified random sample displayed strong decrements in performance scores whereas no such age effect was seen in the educationally balanced sample.

The Schaie and Green studies, together with other similar findings, indicate that much of the cognitive loss in late middle life previously considered a result of "normal" aging may be preventable.[35] The increasing variability in cognitive capacity with advancing age and the likelihood that age-associated declines may be reversible is suggested by recent studies conducted by Schaie and Willis.[36] In a longitudinal study these investigators divided participants into those with a clear pattern of decline in fluid intelligence with advancing age and those whose performance was stable. After five training sessions, cognitive functioning among the individuals who were previously declining substantially improved.

Importance of Transitions in Physical and Psychosocial Status

The marked variability in functional capability and physiologic status and the uncertain link between physiologic changes with advancing age, their functional consequences, and eventual development of disease underline the importance of an approach to the elderly which includes analyses of the transition from one functional or physiologic state to another. Of particular interest in this regard is the dependency of these transitions on factors such as disease, life-style, and change in psychosocial supports. It is inadequate to focus only on mortality, or even morbidity or health care utilization, and increasingly important to evaluate the factors regulating the transition from successful to usual aging.

Health Promotion and Disease Prevention in Older Persons

As recently as a decade ago it seemed paradoxical to speak of health promotion and disease prevention in old age. However, the dramatic longevity revolution engenders the possibility of previously unimagined numbers of frail, infirm, elderly individuals living to advanced old age. The initial claim that as mortality declines morbidity will also decline has recently been challenged by studies suggesting that the increased life span of the "old-old" is not accompanied by decreased morbidity and might actually result in more dramatic increases in the need for health care.[37] With this in mind, it is clear that our attention should focus not on life span but on health span and improving the health status of the elderly.

Attempts to improve the quality of old age require an understanding of the risk factors for common deseases in older persons and the efficacy of strategies to decrease the risk of morbidity. Simplistic generalizations from studies of younger and middle-aged adults to older persons are fraught with difficulty. Little can be gained by telling an eighty-five-year-old woman to reduce the cholesterol in her diet in order to prevent premature heart disease! Recent findings indicating that there is no benefit to the treatment of hypertension over age eighty underline the fact that risk factors for common disorders, such as coronary disease and stroke, may be substantially different in the very old than in the young-old or middle-aged populations.[38]

In addition to the fact that traditional risk factors may be modified with advancing age, we must realize that the outcomes, which are the targets of health promotion/disease prevention activities, may also be quite different in older persons than in their younger counterparts. For instance, in elderly populations the traditional targets of health promotion such as cancer, accidents, heart disease, and stroke should be broadened to include two other categories: (1) the transition from usual to successful aging, discussed above, and (2) a variety of geriatric syndromes. These syndromes are common, morbid, expensive, and previously neglected disorders which occur almost exclusively in elderly individuals and which have received little attention with regard to health promotion and disease prevention programs. Included among these disorders are dementia (which has attracted research investment recently—an investment which is paying dramatic dividends), urinary incontinence, acute confusional state, falling, fainting, nutritional impairments, enhanced sensitivity to medication, and the seemingly ubiquitous "failure to thrive."

Primary among consideration of health promotion and disease prevention in the elderly is recognition of the critical importance of functional status.[39] The provision of health care to the elderly should emphasize maintaining *functional capability*. Although most older Americans living in the community are cognitively intact and fully independent in their daily activities, a substantial proportion of elderly patients who are not institutionalized report major activity limitations due to chronic conditions. Major functional impairments are clearly age related within the elderly, increasing from approximately 5 percent of individuals aged sixty-five to seventy-four requiring assistance with basic activities to nearly 35-40 percent by age eighty-five.[40] Even if one maintains functional independence in old age, the risk of becoming frail is still high. For independent persons between the ages of sixty-five and seventy years, "active life expectancy," that portion of the remaining years characterized by independence, represents about 60 percent.[41] This proportion falls to 40 percent at age eighty-five.

A revolutionary increase in life span has already occurred. A corresponding increase in health span, the maintenance of full function as nearly as possible to the end of life, should be the next gerontological goal. The focus on successful aging elucidates that goal for research workers, practitioners, and for older men and women themselves.

Rationing of Health Care for Older Persons?

A consensus that health care costs must be "contained" developed in the mid-1980s among federal policy-makers concerned with Medicare and Medicaid financing; insurance companies that reimburse hospital charges which include "cost-shifting" from publicly insured patients; insurance premium payers (especially corporate employers that have been paying increasingly higher insurance premiums); and, apparently, the U.S. population in general.[42] As governmental and corporate entities that pay an overwhelming proportion of U.S. health care expenditures attempt to limit their financial obligations, concern has emerged that acute health care will be increasingly rationed.

Expenditures on health care for the aging have been a central theme in many expressions of concern regarding the allocation of U.S. health care resources. There have been repeated public discussions of the high proportion of Medicare that is expended on persons who are in their last year of life.[43] Biomedical ethicists have generated principles of equity to undergird "justice between age groups" in the distribution of health care resources.[44] And conferences have been assembled to address explicitly the issue of "Should medical care be rationed by age?"[45]

It is not surprising that aging would emerge as a central theme in this fevered contemporary milieu of concerns about health care costs. Among the many public and private initiatives to control costs the most widely publicized and far-reaching have been changes in reimbursement procedures under Medicare, which insures all persons aged sixty-five and older. Also, as indicated earlier in this chapter, persons aged sixty-five and older, now 12 percent of the population, account for one-third—presently $142 billion —of annual health care expenditures in the United States.[46] Simple extrapolations from present expenditure patterns and from demographic projections of future growth in the number and proportion of Americans who will be in this age group emphasize the portents of an aging population for both acute and nonacute health care expenditures.

Nonetheless, is there any reason why physicians should change their customary decision-making frameworks regarding the allocation of acute care resources to older patients? Even if physicians somehow were able to feel ethically comfortable with a framework that weights old age more heavily than usual as a criterion for modifying decisions to save lives, would they be able to save a significant amount of health care resources? The answers to these questions appears to be no!

Aging and the Costs of Dying

One practical way to begin to answer such questions is to look at the best available data, which have been summarized by Scitovsky, regarding Medicare expenditures on patients who have lived and died during a twelve-month period.[47] To be sure, there are limitations on such studies. They are retrospective rather than prospective, do not follow through longitudinally with the patients who lived beyond the twelve-month period, and include the approximately 8 percent of Medicare-eligible persons who are not aged sixty-five and older. Moreover, they only provide reimbursement data for services covered by Medicare, not total expenses associated with Medicare services. Consequently, they omit money spent on such items as deductibles and co-payments, drugs, and about 97 percent of payments made to nursing homes. But on balance there is no reason to conclude that these studies are biased either in the direction of understating expenses for those patients who died or those who survived, or that persons under age sixty-five but who are eligible for Medicare because of disability or end-stage renal disease skew the aggregate results. And most to the point, well over 90 percent of the patients in the studies were aged sixty-five and over.

Scitovsky has analytically summarized four such Medicare studies. They all show the same general trends and relationships, although their absolute figures differ slightly. Consequently, the study most worth examining with respect to the issues raised above is the latest, most detailed, and sophisticated, published by Lubitz and Prihoda in 1984, dealing with Medicare expenditures for the year 1978.[48]

This study substantiates many recent statements concerning the high proportion of Medicare funds expended on persons who are in their last year of life. It found that 5.9 percent of Medicare enrollees who died within the year accounted for 27.9 percent of Medicare expenditures for the year. In 1985, in which the total Medicare expenditure was $72 billion,[49] this would mean that about $20 billion in Medicare expenditures was expended on about 6 percent of Medicare eligibles who died. This and the other Medicare studies also make it clear that decedents are more likely than survivors to be hospitalized and reimbursed by Medicare, and that per capita Medicare reimbursements for hospital care are more than seven times higher for decedents than survivors. The good news, of course, would be that Medicare spends more than 2.5 times as much —presently about $52 billion—among the 94 percent of Medicare eligibles who survive.

How Costly Are High-Cost Decedents?

Suppose it were possible, both clinically and ethically, to identify prospectively those Medicare patients who will die within the year, choose not to treat them aggressively, and thereby save "unnecessary health care costs?" How much would be saved in terms of Medicare resources?

A key to answering this question lies in the distribution of reimbursements among decedents. That is, if one were to implement such a framework for clinical decision-making, one would want to begin with the exceptionally high-cost decedents.

The Lubitz and Prihoda study indicated that a relatively small number and percentage of patients sharply affect the average and total costs of reimbursement for care in the last year of life. It found that in 1978 only 3 percent of Medicare-eligible decedents had reimbursements of $20,000 or more, and only 1 percent had reimbursements of $30,000 or more. A parallel study of Medicare enrollees in Colorado in the same year yielded very similar distributions of high-cost reimbursements.[50]

Nationally, the 1 percent of decedents for whom reimbursements were $30,000 or more in 1978 accounted for 1.1 percent of Medicare expenditures for the year or, in 1985 terms, $792 million. The 3 percent of decedents at $20,000 or more accounted for 3.5 percent or, in 1985 terms, $2.52 billion.

In the context of 1985, in which national health care expenditures were $425 billion, such amounts seem negligible. But are they in some sense wasted and/or unnecessary?

Can High Costs on Decedents Be Deemed "Wasted" or "Unnecessary"?

The issue of waste can be addressed by comparing high-cost decedents with high-cost survivors. The Lubitz and Prihoda study found 49,000 Medicare enrollees who received reimbursements of $20,000 or more during 1978. Of these, 24,000 (accounting for 3.5 percent of Medicare reimbursements) died, and 25,000 (accounting for 3.6 percent of Medicare reimbursements) survived. Similarly, 5,000 decedents had reimbursements of $30,000 or more (1.1 percent of Medicare), but an equal number of survivors (5,000) had such reimbursements (also 1.1 percent of Medicare). In other words, almost exactly the same amounts were spent on high-cost Medicare patients who survived as were spent on decedents. In light of preoccupations with cost containment, perhaps some persons would regard it to have been important, retrospectively, to have saved $2.52 billion or even $792 million by not treating aggressively the high-cost patients who died.

But since prospective distinctions between survivors and decedents are often problematic—especially in cases that are likely to involve high costs—how could one operationalize a cost-containment policy that would try to single out prospectively the high-cost patients who are almost certainly going to die within the year? Even if it were ethically palatable?

Predicting death far in advance—twelve, five, or three months in advance—with a high degree of certainty is beyond the present state-of-art in medicine. As Scitovsky notes, "The main exceptions are cancer patients for whom a prognosis of death can be made with reasonable accuracy beyond a certain point in the course of their disease; and it is no accident that hospice programs serve primarily such patients."[51] In short, on the basis of available evidence, one cannot use the high probability that treatment of a patient will incur large costs as an indicator of a probable waste of health care resources. To do so would throw the survivors into the same "wastebasket" with the decedents.

Will Population Aging Change Allocation Patterns?

There are no practical means or reasons for physicians to change their customary clinical decision-making frameworks regarding the allocation of health care resources to older persons. And there is no apparent reason to alter the traditional ethical principles of the medical profession. What implications, then, can be drawn from the many expressions of concern about the need to confront issues of more explicit and extensive health care rationing—weighting old age more heavily as a criterion—than experienced since the implementation of Medicare and Medicaid two decades ago?

Certainly the basis for concern about rationing on the basis of old age is not a scarcity of health care resources. Health care resources are expanding, not shrinking. In 1985 health care spending in the United States increased 8.9 percent even though, due to slower price inflation, this was the lowest annual growth in two decades.[52]

Nor can the basis for concern among the general public be the fierce competition among health care providers that has been brought about by cost containment measures that have changed the prices, sources, and mechanisms of payment for health care. For those who are winning in the competition, resources are plentiful, and they are willing to transcend traditional barriers to undertake greater than ever acute health care interventions, even for persons aged seventy-five and over.[53] For the providers who are losing, resources are scarce. It is for their customers —patients dependent upon public insurance and the medically indigent with no insurance—that resources are scarce, and for whom medical care is rationed. This has been the case traditionally, and allocation patterns may remain much as they have been.

A possible implication of the concern about rationing is that the challenges of an aging population have provided a metaphor for our society to discuss the issues of allocation or "distributive justice" of health care resources more openly than in the past. We are now considering issues of "justice between age groups" after several decades of experiencing the societal luxury of pretending that physicians and their associates were doing everything they could for everyone.

The establishment of Medicare and Medicaid in 1965 largely eliminated the phenomenon of "charity cases" by providing public reimbursement for the care of indigent patients and promoting the goals of equal care and equal access to care for all. But as Medicare and Medicaid cutbacks have accelerated cost-shifting from the medically indigent to those who have other insurance or can pay out of pocket—and as insurance companies, insurance premium payers, out-of-pocket payers, and state governments have reacted by resisting cost-shifting—the luxury of the pretense of equal access and equal care is eroding.

Now that the pretense is eroding, perhaps "justice between age groups" is a more convenient and comfortable metaphor for discussing the allocation patterns in our health care arena than "justice between rich and poor." If we put aside our preoccupation with Medicare and "the geriatric imperative," we can recognize that it is the capacity of patients to pay for charges—out of pocket or through third-party reimbursements—that has a great deal to do with the allocation of care.

Maybe the concern about old-age-based rationing is justified. But what would happen if Medicare coverage became sharply reduced, means-tested, or totally eliminated? Some older persons would be able to pay out of pocket for all the high-quality care they need and want, and many more would be able to pay the premiums that would insure most of the costs of acute care. Near-poor and poor older persons would be left in the same position as medically indigent persons of all ages. Viewed in this light, rationing and its tacit judgments regarding the worthiness of human lives might mean, simply, a continuation of the traditional American style of justice: distribution of health care resources—as well as, for example, educational resources—on the basis of social and economic class.

The increasing older population will certainly play a substantial role in shaping organizations, financing and delivery mechanisms in the health care arena, as well as in the practice of medicine. But there is no reason to expect that population aging will change America's long-standing tradition of allocating health care and other societal resources among its citizens.

Notes

1. A. Somers and D. Fabian, eds., *The Geriatric Imperative: An Introduction to Gerontology and Clinical Geriatrics* (New York: Appleton-Century-Crofts, 1981).

2. G. C. Myers, "The Aging of Populations," in R. H. Binstock, W-S Chow, and J. H. Schulz, eds., *International Perspectives on Aging: Population and Policy Challenges* (New York: United Nations Fund for Population Activities, 1982); and U.S. Senate Special Committee on Aging, *Developments in Aging: 1985, Vol. 3* (Washington, D.C.: GPO, 1986).

3. Committee on an Aging Society/Institute of Medicine and National Research Council, *Health in an Older Society* (Washington, D.C.: National Academy Press, 1985); and "The Aging Society," *Daedalus, Journal of the American Academy of Arts and Sciences* 115 (1986):1–395.

4. U. S. Senate Special Committee on Aging, *Developments in Aging*.

5. U.S. Senate Special Committee on Aging, *Aging America: Trends and Projec-*

tions—1985–86 Edition (Washington, D.C.: American Association of Retired Persons, 1986).

6. U. S. Senate Special Committee on Aging, *Developments in Aging.*

7. M. Gornick et al., "Twenty Years of Medicare and Medicaid: Covered Populations, Use of Benefits, and Program Expenditures," *Health Care Financing Review,* annual supplement (1985):13–59.

8. E. N. Gruenberg, "The Failures of Success," *Milbank Memorial Fund Quarterly/Health and Society* 55 (1977):3–24; and E. L. Schneider and J. A. Brody, "Aging, Natural Death, and the Compression of Morbidity: Another View," *New England Journal of Medicine* 309 (1983):854–856.

9. U.S. Senate Special Committee, *Aging America.*

10. U.S. Senate Special Committee, *Aging America.*

11. Committee on an Aging Society, *Health in an Older Society.*

12. Schneider and Brody, "Aging, Natural Death: Another View"; J. F. Fries, "Aging, Natural Death, and the Compression of Morbidity," *New England Journal of Medicine* 303 (1980):130–135; J. F. Fries, "An Introduction to the Compression of Morbidity," *Gerontologica Critica* (in press); E. L. Schneider and J. M. Guralnik, "The Compression of Morbidity: A Dream Which May Come True, Someday!" *Gerontologica Critica* (in press); and R. H. Binstock, "Exhortatory and Scholarly Approaches to the Compression of Morbidity: A Commentary on Fries and Schneider/Guralnik," *Gerontologica Critica* (in press).

13. H. B. Brotman, *Every Ninth American: An Analysis for the Chairman of the Select Committee on Aging, U.S. House of Representatives* (Washington, D.C.: GPO, 1982).

14. J. A. Weintraub and B. A. Burt, "Oral Health Status in the United States: Tooth Loss and Edentulism," *Journal of Dental Education* 49 (1985):368–376.

15. U.S. Senate Special Committee, *Aging America.*

16. U.S. Senate Special Committee, *Aging America.*

17. J. W. Rowe, "Health Care of the Elderly," *New England Journal of Medicine* 312 (1985): 827–835; and N. W. Shock et al., *Normal Human Aging: The Baltimore Longitudinal Study of Aging* (Washington, D.C.: U.S. Department of Health and Human Services, 1984).

18. Rowe, "Health Care of the Elderly." Shock et al., *Normal Human Aging;* and J. W. Rowe, "Clinical Research in Aging: Strategies and Directions," *New England Journal of Medicine* 297 (1977):1332–1336.

19. K. L. Minaker, G. S. Meneilly, and J. W. Rowe, "Endocrine Systems," in C. E. Finch and E. L. Schneider, eds., *Handbook of the Biology of Aging* (New York: Van Nostrand Reinhold, 1985), p. 437.

20. M. B. Davidson, "The Effects of Aging on Carbohydrate Metabolism," *Metabolism* 28 (1979):688–705.

21. International Collaborative Group on Asymptomatic Hyperglycemia and Coronary Heart Disease, *Journal of Chronic Disease* 32 (1979): 11--12.

22. P. Ducimetiere et al., "Relationship of Plasma Insulin Levels to the Incidence of Myocardial Infarction and Coronary Heart Disease Mortality in a Middle Aged Population," *Diabetologia* 19 (1980):205; K. Pyorala, *Diabetes Care* 2 (1979):131; and T. A. Welborn and K. Wearne, "Coronary Heart Disease, Inci-

dence and Cardiovascular Mortality in Busselton with Reference to Glucose and Insulin Concentrations," *Diabetes Care* 2 (1979):154.

23. M. S. Greenfield et al., "Effect of Age on Plasma Triglyceride Concentrations in Man," *Metabolism* 29 (1980):1095; L. A. Carlson and L. E. Bottinger, "Ischemic Heart Disease in Relation to Fasting Value of Plasma Triglycerides and Cholesterol," Stockholm Prospective Study, *Lancet* 1 (1972):865; and I. Zavaroni et al., "Evidence for an Independent Relationship between Plasma, Insulin, and Concentration of High Density Lipoprotein Cholesterol and Triglyceride," *Atherosclerosis* 55 (1985):259.

24. I. Zavaroni et al., "Effect of Age and Environmental Factors on Glucose Tolerance and Insulin Secretion in a Worker Population," *Journal of the American Geratric Society* 34 (1986):271–275.

25. C. B. Hollenbeck et al., "Effect of Habitual Physical Activity on Regulation of Insulin-Stimulated Glucose Disposal in Older Males," *Journal of the American Geratric Society* 33 (1985):273–277.

26. G. M. Reaven and E. P. Reaven, "Age, Glucose Intolerance and Non-Insulin Dependent Diabetes Mellitus," *Journal of the American Geratric Society* 33 (1985):286–287.

27. D. E. James, E. W. Kraegen, and D. J. Chisholm, "Effect of Exercise Training on Whole-Body Insulin Sensitivity and Responsiveness," *Journal of Applied Physiology* 56 (1984):1217; D. L. Seals et al., "Glucose Tolerance in Young and Older Athletes and Sedentary Men," *Journal of Applied Physiology* 56 (1984):1521; and R. P. Tonino et al., "Effect of Physical Training on the Insulin Resistance of Aging," *Clinical Research* 34 (1986):557A.

28. B. L. Briggs and L. J. Melton, "Involutional Osteoporosis," *New England Journal of Medicine* 314 (1986):1676–1685.

29. Briggs and Melton, "Involutional Osteoporosis."

30. E. Seeman et al., "Risk Factors for Spinal Osteoporosis in Men," *American Journal of Medicine* 75 (1983):977–983; D. D. Bikle et al., "Bone Disease and Alcohol Abuse," *Annals of Internal Medicine* 103 (1982):42–48; M. A. Adena and H. G. Gallagher, "Risk Factors for Osteoporosis," *Annals of Human Biology* 9 (1982):121; and H. Jick, J. Porter, and A. S. Morrison, "Relation Between Smoking and Age of Natural Menopause," *Lancet* 1 (1983):1354–1355.

31. J. F. Aloia et al., "Prevention of Involutional Bone Loss by Exercise," *Annals of Internal Medicine* 89 (1978):356–358; B. Krolner et al., "Physical Exercise as Prophylaxis Against Involutional Vertebral Bone Loss: A Control Trial," *Clinical Science* 64 (1983):541–546; and E. L. Smith, W. Reddan, and P. E. Smith, "Physical Activity and Calcium Modalities for Bone Mineral Increase in Aged Women," *Medical Science Sports Exercise* 13 (1981):60–64.

32. G. Labouvie-Vief, "Intelligence and Cognition," in J. E. Birren and K. W. Shaie, eds., *Handbook of the Psychology of Aging* (New York: Van Nostrand Reinhold, 1985), p. 500–530.

33. K. W. Schaie and G. Labouvie-Vief, "Generational Versus Ontogenetic Components of Change in Adult Cognitive Behavior: A Fourteen Year Cross Sequential Study," *Developmental Psychology* 10 (1974):305–320.

34. R. F. Green, "Age-Intelligence Relationships Between Ages 16 and 64. A Rising Trend," *Developmental Psychology* 1 (1969):618–627.

35. Labouvie-Vief, "Intelligence and Cognition."

36. K. W. Schaie and S. Willis, "Can Decline in Adult Intellectual Functioning be Reversed?" *Developmental Psychology* 22 (1986):223.

37. Schneider and Brody, "Aging, Natural Death: Another View."

38. A. Amery et al., "Efficacy of Antihypertensive Drug Treatment According to Age, Sex, Blood Pressure, and Previous Cardiovascular Disease in Patients over the Age of 60," *Lancet* 2 (1986):589-592.

39. Rowe, "Health Care of the Elderly."

40. National Center for Health Statistics, *Americans Needing Help to Function at Home* (Hyattsville, Md.: Public Health Service, September 14, 1983).

41. S. Katz et al., "Active Life Expectancy," *New England Journal of Medicine* 309 (1983):1218–1224.

42. Lou Harris and Associates, Inc., *The Equitable Health Care Survey* (Washington, D.C.: Lou Harris and Associates, 1983).

43. J. Schulte, "Terminal Patients Deplete Medicare, Greenspan Says," *Dallas Morning News*, 26 April 1983, p. 1.

44. N. Daniels, "Justice Between Age Groups: Am I My Parents' Keeper?" *Milbank Memorial Fund Quarterly/Health and Society* 61 (1983):489--522.

45. T. M. Smeeding et al., eds., *Should Medical Care Be Rationed by Age?* (Totowa, N. J.: Rowman & Littlefield, forthcoming).

46. D. R. Waldo, K. R. Levit, and H. Lazenby, "National Health Expenditures, 1985," *Health Care Financing Review* 8 (1986):1–21.

47. A. A. Scitovsky, "'The High Cost of Dying': What Do the the Data Show?" *Milbank Memorial Fund Quarterly/Health and Society* 62 (1984):591–608.

48. J. Lubitz and R. Prihoda, "The Use and Costs of Medicare Services in the Last Two Years of Life," *Health Care Financing Review* 5 (1984):117–131.

49. Waldo et al., "National Health Expenditures, 1985."

50. N. McCall, "Utilization and Costs of Medicare Services by Beneficiaries in Their Last Year of Life," *Medical Care* 22 (1984):329–342.

51. Scitovsky, "High Cost of Dying."

52. Waldo et al., "National Health Expenditures, 1985." 53. R. Koenig, "As Liver Transplants Grow More Common, Ethical Issues Multiply: By Operating on the Elderly, Thomas Starzl Steps Up Patient Selection Debate," *Wall Street Journal*, 14 October 1986, p. 1.

53. R. Koenig, "As Liver Transplants Grow More Common, Ethical Issues Multiply: By Operating on the Elderly, Thomas Starzl Steps Up Patient Selection Debate," *Wall Street Journal*, 14 October 1986, p. 1.

7

The New Genetics and the Future Practice of Medicine

Leon E. Rosenberg

Introduction

Genetics, a young science and an even younger clinical specialty, has become a household word. It is virtually impossible to read a newspaper or magazine or to turn on the radio or television set without encountering something about genetics. Such accounts portray an exciting array of advances. One day this progress involves the use of recombinant DNA (rDNA) technology to produce unlimited amounts of previously scarce and medically useful hormones such as insulin and growth hormone. The next day we learn that the genes for Huntington's disease and cystic fibrosis have been mapped to chromosome 4 and chromosome 7, respectively, thereby providing new approaches to the diagnosis, and ultimately the treatment and/or prevention of these dread diseases. On a third day we find out that all normal human cells contain genes (proto-oncogenes) which control cell growth and which, when rearranged or mutated, can lead to cancer (oncogenes).

But descriptions of scientific progress and clinical promise are not, by any means, all that genetics calls forth.[1] The Vatican brands as immoral "alternative" means of reproduction such as artificial insemination or in vitro fertilization which may serve as options for couples at risk of having children with genetic diseases.[2] The Surgeon General of the United States is reported to have called prenatal diagnosis of genetic disease a "search and destroy mission" because it leads, in a very small fraction of cases, to abortion. Individuals and groups seek to halt all work aimed at human gene therapy for fear that the technology will lead first to the creation of Frankenstein-like monsters and ultimately to the destruction of man as a species.[3] Biotechnology companies spring up by the hundreds, many fashioned by university scientists who find no conflict of interest or commitment in adding the personal profit motive to the others which drive their careers.[4]

Historical Perspective

This public discussion of genetics—from the elementary school classroom to the corporate boardroom—is unprecedented in the history of the biological or medical sciences. It is also a very recent phenomenon. The discovery of the laws of dominant and recessive inheritance of single factors (now called genes) by Mendel in the 1860s went unnoticed for forty years as did Garrod's formulation in 1900 of biochemical individuality (through his study of several rare, human "inborn errors of metabolism"). Even the discovery by Avery, McLeod, and McCarty (1944) that DNA was the "transforming principle" in bacteria (i.e., that genes are made of DNA) received little attention until Beadle and Tatum deduced, at about the same time, that genes act by coding for proteins (the one gene-one enzyme hypothesis). Genetics came of age when Watson and Crick (1953) predicted that all of the fundamental properties of DNA could be accounted for by a double helical conformation of its purine and pyrimidine bases, its sugars, and its phosphate groups. It was, in truth, this brilliant formulation of the structure of DNA—this ultimate reduction of unfathomable biological complexity into startling, chemical simplicity—that drew to the field in turn a growing band of molecular biologists, clinicians, and ethicists, each group convinced that, for good or bad, genetics was to have a profound impact on our society because it promised to offer mankind a powerful understanding of itself and its relationship to all other living creatures.

The New Genetics

The discovery of rDNA technology in the early 1970s by Cohen and Boyer[5] was to the application of genetics what the formulation of the double helix had been to the fundamental understanding of gene structure and function. The ability to propagate any gene, regardless of origin, by recombining it with simple molecules (plasmids or viruses) designed to serve merely as growth vehicles (or vectors), gave enormous impetus to the scientists' ability to identify, localize, map, sequence, and understand genes. rDNA technology constituted a paradigm shift in methodology; it made possible, quickly, advances hitherto only speculated or fretted about. Suddenly, "genetic engineering" (a term coined in 1965 by Hotchkiss in reference to strategies by which genetically determined characteristics could be added to cells or organisms that did not possess them[6]) was a reality. Suddenly, cloning any gene was essentially trivial, albeit laborious, as was getting it to be expressed by inserting it (transfection) into cells in culture. Suddenly, genes and chromosomes could be manipulated like pieces of string, capable of being cut up and rejoined (by highly specific chemical "scissors" proteins called restriction enzymes) so as to ask questions about one or another "piece" by studying it in isolation. Suddenly, the ability to map and order the approximately 10,000-100,000 genes in the human genome was feasible. In fact, it was this latter notion which led Comings[7] to coin the term "new genetics" to describe a seminal paper written by Botstein et al.[8] in which they demonstrated that the human genome could be mapped by using restriction enzymes to identify normal variations in the genome. These variations are called restriction fragment length polymorphisms or RFLPs. Their identification has simplified genetic linkage analysis in man so that it is no longer the arcane tool of a mathematically sophisticated few.

Impact on Society

Throughout history, from the ancient discovery of fire to the modern discovery of atomic energy, profound scientific discoveries have always engendered powerful societal debates. Looked at in this way, we should not be surprised that many of the applications resulting from discoveries in genetics have provoked major controversy. When it became clear in the 1940s and 1950s that certain genetic diseases were clustered in certain ethnic groups—like β-thalassemia in Italians, Tay-Sachs disease in Ashkenazi Jews, and sickle-cell anemia in blacks—there were those who feared that such information would be used to justify "eugenic" horrors such as the genocidal holocaust perpetrated by Hitler. When it was learned in the 1960s that diagnosing phenylketonuria in newborns could be followed by dietary therapy capable of preventing the severe mental retardation characteristic of this disease and allowing near normal growth, development, and procreation, there were those who opposed treatment of such biologically imperfect individuals because they and their progeny would "pollute" the human gene pool. When it was shown in the 1970s that prenatal diagnosis of lethal genetic disorders such as trisomy 13 or anencephaly was feasible and could offer parents the choice of continuing or terminating such pregnancies, there were those who demanded that this technology be banned lest we create a world in which only perfect, sex-selected offspring would be accepted.

When looked at with this historical perspective, it is not surprising that the real and imaginary ethical dilemmas presented by the rDNA-driven new genetics have been discussed from its inception. What is unique is that these societal debates have occurred *before* the technologies have been widely used. The 1975 Asilomar Conference, organized by scientists when rDNA technology was still embryonic in use, called for a moratorium on laboratory experiments using rDNA technology until stringent experimental guidelines could be promulgated by a national advisory committee.[9] Similarly, the President's Commission for the Study of Ethical Problems in Medicine and Biomedical and Behavioral Research scrutinized and gave its support to somatic cell gene therapy in man years ahead of the development of the medical technology for such an approach.[10] Such conferences and commissions have not satisfied everyone. In truth, there is nothing except a complete ban on all inquiry in this area that will satisfy those fearful that genetics will destroy mankind by unlocking the ultimate mysteries of our species. Fortunately, such prohibitions will not be enacted by our society because most people see that the actual and potential benefits of this field far outweigh the risks.

Clinical Applications

It is the potential and present applications of the new genetics to clinical medicine which I now wish to address. These will be in each of the four major areas of clinical understanding: etiology and pathogenesis, diagnosis, treatment, and prevention.

Etiology and Pathogenesis

The new genetics will be a spectacular catalyst for unraveling the mysteries of the cause and mechanism of diseases. Its impact—potential and immediate—for dealing with genetic diseases is particularly exciting, since genetic disorders have a major impact on human health. If we accept the definition of the term "genetic disease" as a disorder for which a variant DNA sequence is a major determinant resulting in impairment, disability, or handicap, three major categories of genetic diseases are recognizable. The first category—and the least well understood—is made up of a large number of conditions called multifactorial traits. Prime examples of such conditions are neural tube defects, congenital heart lesions, juvenile onset diabetes mellitus, and essential hypertension. Multifactorial traits result from complex interactions between one or more genes and the environment. Such conditions cluster in families but are not inherited as simple Mendelian dominant or recessive traits. The next category of genetic disease—chromosomal abnormalities—is made up of disorders like Down's syndrome, Fragile X syndrome, and Turner syndrome in which there is a microscopically identifiable increase or decrease in the total mass of chromosomal material in the cell. Since each chromosome carries thousands of genes, such chromosomal abnormalities probably produce their major, sometimes lethal, clinical consequences by affecting many systems and reactions. The third major category of genetic disease is the single gene defects such as cystic fibrosis, sickle-cell anemia, familial hypercholesterolemia, and muscular dystrophy. These disorders are inherited as autosomal or X-linked dominant or recessive traits depending on the location and function of the specific gene in question. We understand many disorders in this category in considerable molecular and cellular detail. All genetic disorders have an overall incidence in liveborn babies in excess of 6 percent—the multifactorial traits account for more than half. Multifactorial traits are responsible for nearly one-third of all admissions to pediatric inpatient services and a like fraction of childhood deaths. Chromosomal abnormalities are thought to be responsible for one-half of all spontaneous abortions indicating that what we see at birth is the "tip of the iceberg" of these conditions. More than 2,000 different single gene defects are known and, though most of these disorders are individually rare, their collective impact is profound particularly because of the high fraction of these disorders which lead to early death, reproductive incapacity, or developmental retardation. Currently, only 300 out of more than 3,000 inherited disorders due to single gene defects are understood sufficiently to lend themselves to rapid scrutiny using new genetic strategies, but each week's journals inform us that the biochemical and molecular basis for another inherited disease has been elucidated through molecular genetic techniques.

We can predict safely that in the near future the number of disorders we will have mastered, because of recombinant DNA technology and its attendant applications in cell biology and structural biology, will continue to increase. Already much has been learned about specific inherited diseases. The work being done on the thalassemias is exemplary of how this technology is sharpening our focus.[11] Before this new biotechnology was available, children in many Mediterranean countries were diagnosed as having β-thalassemia, a severe and widespread anemia known to result from an inherited defect in these affected children's β-globin gene. Now, with the help of new genetic technologies, we know that β-thalassemia is not one but a family of closely related disorders, all of which result in anemia. Because β-thalassemia is the most common and most prevalent blood disorder in the world, and because many of the countries in which thalassemia is found are poor, and because thalassemic patients require blood transfusions throughout their lifetimes, the implications for understanding better this disorder are far-reaching.[12] The new biotechnology has helped us measure how great the problems are for dealing humanely and effectively with this one disease constellation.

However complex and heterogeneous β-thalassemia turns out to be in molecular terms, studying its etiology has been approached using a traditional strategy. That is, first the physiologic derangement was recognized, next the abnormal gene product (protein or enzyme) was identified, and, finally, the precise genetic locus and mutation were uncovered. This strategy may be called "forward" genetics, and its use will be accelerated dramatically by new genetic technologies. From it we will learn which inborn errors result from nucleotide base insertions, deletions, and substitutions. From it we will find out which inherited disorders are caused by a single mutation (e.g., sickle-cell anemia) and which are as heterogeneous as the thalassemias. For more than 90 percent of all inherited disorders, however, we have not ascertained what the specific influential gene product is. Because such conditions are inherited as Mendelian recessive, dominant, or X-linked traits, we have long known that they were caused by defects at a single genetic locus, but our ignorance of the precise locus of these aberrations has greatly hampered our ability to understand, as well as to diagnose and to treat them. It is these disorders—including such common and lethal conditions as cystic fibrosis,[13] muscular dystrophy,[14] and Huntington's disease[15]—which are already being approached by "reverse" genetic strategies spawned by the new genetics. In these instances, anonymous pieces of human DNA, prepared by cutting up a portion of the entire genome with restriction enzymes to make a library from the pieces, have been used to identify RFLP linkage markers located close enough to "track" the disease being investigated. Identifying a useful marker determines the gene's chromosomal location. Next, it is necessary to "walk" from the linkage marker toward the specific disease locus by using a series of differently spliced, ordered, marker probes. This is the state of the field at present, but in the near future, the precise locus will be identified and its DNA sequenced to deduce the gene product it encodes. Then, these predictions based on DNA analysis alone will be confirmed by studies examining gene expression in intact cells or fractions therefrom.

Perhaps it is even more dramatic to begin to witness the applicability of this new genetic technology on less well understood human diseases. Within the past few months, for example, it has been demonstrated that a familial form of Alzheimer's disease has been mapped to a locus on chromosome 21[16] and familial forms of manic-depressive illness to the X chromosome and to chromosome 11.[17] These studies prove incontrovertibly that certain forms of each of these major illnesses will ultimately be traced to single gene products; they herald the approach which will be used to identify genetic loci and their corresponding products. As importantly, these studies demonstrate that, in the case of manic-depressive illness, what may appear to be a single clinical phenotype actually can be subdivided into several genetically distinct entities. Such heterogeneity will ultimately lead to a more detailed understanding of pathogenesis.

In the future, this approach will yield information concerning the etiology of schizophrenia, diabetes, hypertension, and coronary heart disease—major illnesses whose multifactorial bases have been surmised from previous work but whose dissection into specific entities has not been realized to date. Ultimately, we will learn that each of these syndromes is a collection of many different disorders, some with major genetic components in their etiology, some with minor. An exciting illustration of this point concerns recent findings in individuals with coronary heart disease, a major cause of death in this country. The Nobel Prize-winning work of Brown and Goldstein demonstrated that one form of coronary disease resulting from hypercholesterolemia is due to the dysfunction of the cell surface receptor which allows circulating cholesterol to enter cells.[18] More recent work from their laboratory, using rDNA technology, has again defined the heterogeneous nature for this well-characterized condition. Other groups are now using similar technologies to define other etiologic entities. Further, in the same way that patients with a receptor defect have been aided by particular drugs or diets aimed at lowering their blood cholesterol, so will definition of new pathogenetic entities within the coronary artery disease syndrome lead to more effective management regimens, tailor-made to the specific genetic lesion identified.

The impact of these new genetic approaches on disease classification, nosology, and understanding will nowhere be greater than in the field of cancer research. Although a large body of information on such topics as chemical carcinogenesis, chromosomal rearrangement in malignant cells, transforming retroviruses, and Mendelian disorders in man predisposing to malignancy has been amassed during the past century, progress toward a fundamental understanding of the process(es) by which cells become malignant has been disappointingly slow. Very recently, however, and largely because of the application of new genetic technologies, unifying hypotheses have emerged which related neoplasia to the malfunction of a relatively small number of cancer-causing genes called oncogenes.[19] These genes, perhaps thirty to fifty in number, normally code for a variety of products found in the nucleus, the cytoplasm, and the membranes of normal cells. They almost surely are critical factors in controlling normal cell growth and differentiation. When one (or perhaps more) of these oncogenes becomes dysfunctional, either because it undergoes point mutations, becomes amplified (more than one copy per chromosome), or gets moved to a new location due to chromosomal breakage and rearrangement, it no longer functions properly. Such gene malfunction then triggers, in ways yet obscure, cellular transformation ultimately leading to malignancy. Support for this model has come from many laboratories working with a variety of tumors affecting lung, bladder, bowel, brain, lymph nodes, and circulating blood cells. It is safe to predict that present and future efforts will not only solve the riddle of cancer cell formation, but may also provide insights into such other crucial issues as why some tumors metastasize and why some become resistant to drug therapy or radiation treatment.

Diagnosis

Among the most important facets of technology upon which the new genetics has been built is the ability to select a single fragment of DNA from a complex mixture of DNA fragments. This technology involves the following steps: isolation of DNA from any cell or tissue source; cutting up the DNA by restriction endonuclease enzymes; separation of the DNA fragments according to size using electrophoresis; and identification of a single DNA segment by hybridizing (binding) to it an homologous small segment of highly purified, isotopically or chemically labeled DNA known as a "probe." With only minor variations, this hybridization analysis is carried out the same way regardless of the probe employed. Thus, its use is limited only by the number of available probes. Because genes, coding for all sorts of proteins, are being cloned rapidly today, a large repertoire of probes of striking specificity is being produced; this probe bank will quickly increase in range and value. In clinical terms this means that in the offing is a major new diagnostic capability whose operational simplicity, versatility, and broad applications makes it particularly promising.

In the not very distant future, I believe this technology will revolutionize testing in clinical laboratories. As we learn more about the specific genes responsible for the very large number of genetic diseases in man, probes will be developed for each disorder based on the chemical "signature" of the gene or disease. Disease-specific probes have already been developed for such disorders as sickle-cell anemia in which the exact nature of the mutation is known. Probes with this degree of specificity are few in number at present because we understand currently only a handful of diseases at this level of detail. For many other conditions, however, we have probes corresponding to the locus at which the disease-causing mutation has occurred (as in phenylketonuria, hemophilia, urea cycle disorders) or we have anonymous DNA probes closely linked (i.e., that occur nearby) to the disease-related gene. In these instances the hybridization tests are much more laborious because they depend on family studies in which the chromosome bearing the mutation (rather than the precise mutation itself) is sought. This usually means that DNA samples must be isolated from the patient, one or both parents, and a healthy sibling. Such family-based diagnosis is currently conducted in specialized genetics laboratories in medical centers throughout the world. Before long, however, clinical laboratories in major hospitals will also provide this service. This transition from "cottage industry"-based diagnostic capability to centralized facilities will occur in many places over the next decade. It will require that clinicians ordering the tests and technicians performing them understand basic genetic principles in order, first, to obtain samples from appropriate family members and second, to interpret the data accurately.

In my view, however, such hybridization methods will have an even more powerful effect on the diagnosis of infectious diseases than on genetic disorders. Every bacterium, fungus, or virus has a unique DNA composition--its own genetic signature. As we learn more about the development of probes specific for given microorganisms, the kind of hybridization test described above for genetic disorders will come to be useful for the diagnosis of infectious diseases. Currently, a patient suspected of having pneumonia due to the pneumococcus must wait one to two days for a sample of sputum to be collected, stained, and cultured before the organism is identified absolutely. Diagnosing patients suffering from viral pneumonia or other viral illnesses such as herpes or AIDS is more complex because virus growth and isolation takes much longer and requires highly specialized culture conditions. In the future, such bacteriologic diagnosis will be made within a few minutes after the sample of sputum, blood, or cerebrospinal fluid has been subjected to DNA analysis using a probe specific for the suspected bacterium or virus. Rapid determination of the specific pathogen will facilitate expeditious selection and administration of antibiotics. This will shorten the duration of clinical disability in some instances; it will save lives in others—particularly those individuals with fulminant infections (like bacterial meningitis) for whom a single day of imperfect antibiotic selection might be crucial. Can such testing be extended to other rampant illnesses like AIDS, for instance, by replacing current technology based on the presence of antibody to the virus? It is too early to say, but attempts in that direction will surely be made.

Treatment

Recombinant DNA technology will affect treatment of human disease in two quite different ways: through the production of useful reagents and through the insertion of normal genes into cells bearing mutated ones. The former application is already at hand, the latter is not yet ready for clinical trial. Both have important implications for clinical medicine.

Within the past few years, two major proteins—each a hormone—have been mass produced by inserting a human gene into bacteria and allowing these engineered organisms to synthesize the human hormone.[20] Insulin and growth hormone were made available this way. Diabetes and dwarfism are the diseases whose treatment has been changed by the availability of insulin and growth hormone, respectively. The availability of pure human insulin will definitely reduce a significant problem encountered in diabetic patients treated with nonhuman insulins—namely the development of anti-insulin antibodies. Furthermore, it should be possible to prepare a more homogeneous, reproducibly active insulin molecule by laboratory-controlled rDNA technology than by having to rely on batch-purified, animal-derived material.

The treatment of growth hormone deficiency promises to be effected even more dramatically. Currently, growth hormone is obtained in tiny amounts from human pituitary glands at autopsy. The limited amount of hormone made in this way has meant that very few people can be treated. It has meant, too, that in a few cases tragedies have occurred because a few batches of this hormone were contaminated with the slow virus responsible for Jakob-Creutzfeldt disease (which infects the brain). rDNA-derived growth hormone will eliminate both problems but will create at least one important new one; namely, what will be the indications for the use of growth hormone in man? The current restricted supply has meant strict rationing and allocation only to children with severe short stature due to isolated growth hormone deficiency. When the supply of growth hormone is more abundant, it seems likely that parents of children who are merely small but not dwarfed will want their children to receive growth hormone supplements to stimulate growth. It is not clear whether such supplementary use of growth hormone will be effective or whether any ill effects will result therefrom.

In the relatively near future a number of other disorders will be approached using products made by rDNA technology: factor VIII for hemophilia; erythropoietin for certain kinds of anemia; α_1-antitrypsin for its deficiency state; tissue plasminogen activator for thrombotic cardiovascular disease. With the high incidence in our population of thrombotic conditions, the latter application is being watched with particular interest.

The other therapeutic application—gene therapy—requires more detailed discussion. Human gene therapy may be defined as the introduction of a normal functioning human gene into the cells of an individual in which its defective mutant counterpart is active. The purpose of such therapy is to abolish the deleterious clinical consequences resulting from expression of the mutant gene. Let me underscore that human gene therapy has the same ethical goal as all other forms of medical treatment—reduction of human suffering and restoration of health. Sometime in the future we can imagine that a couple who have already had a child with sickle-cell anemia (or a large number of other well-characterized genetic disorders) will be spared the anguish they now suffer when informed, upon the birth of their next child that he/she, too, has this debilitating disease. When gene therapy has become a reality, it will be possible to take cells from the affected child, grow them in culture, insert the correct gene for globin production into them, and finally reintroduce these healthy cells back into the child. These new cells will repopulate the child's bone marrow and produce the normal hemoglobin it was lacking.

The ethical issues here are straightforward. This form of gene therapy is comparable to the current and widely accepted procedure of bone marrow transplantation. The objective of bone marrow transplantation is to insert normal cells into a patient whose cells are defective; the aim of somatic cell gene therapy is to insert normal genes into a patient's cells in which the genes are defective. Such somatic cell gene therapy will have no effect on the human gene pool because no modification of the germ cell has been undertaken; hence the inserted gene cannot be passed on to the patient's offspring.

In theory, gene therapy directed at germ cells, the fertilized oocyte for instance, would appear to have some real advantages. Injecting genes into oocytes of experimental animals is relatively simple and efficient to perform. If successfully accomplished, every cell of the recipient would contain the inserted gene, thus permitting treatment of disorders which affect many different tissues, like cystic fibrosis. However, these advantages are overwhelmed by three problems.[21] First, we currently lack the means to diagnose any disorder in the fertilized oocyte and thereby assure that the embryo, whose risk of being affected may be 1 in 2 (50 percent) or 1 in 4 (25 percent), has the disease in question. Without this capability, which will be difficult to develop and risky to employ, germ line gene therapy is not feasible. Second, studies in which genes have been inserted into mouse oocytes have already demonstrated that major deleterious consequences in the progeny are common, not rare. Third, there is the powerful ethical issue raised by realizing that germ line gene therapy will result in the inserted genes being passed on to the recipient's offspring and to all subsequent generations. For these reasons, human germ line gene therapy cannot and should not be contemplated at this time.

Which kinds of human genetic diseases would be candidates for gene therapy? The answer is that human somatic cell gene therapy could be employed in the forseeable future only for single gene defects because it is only in this category that we have sufficient understanding of the molecular basis of the disease to know which gene should be isolated and inserted. Thus, however promising gene therapy may be, it is potentially applicable only to a very small fraction of patients with genetic diseases.

How close are we to attempting somatic cell gene therapy in man? Answers to that question range widely depending on which expert you poll.[22] Certain steps in the development of therapeutic protocols no longer present a problem, i.e., selection of suitable disease candidates and cloning their respective genes. There is agreement that gene therapy will be tried first in disorders whose primary pathophysiology effects circulating blood cells, because these cells can be removed from and replaced back into the bone marrow without much difficulty. Two prime disease candidates are: defects in globin synthesis, like sickle-cell anemia or β-thalassemia, and disorders like adenosine deaminase deficiency resulting in severe impairment of the immune system. These respective genes have been cloned and studied intensively in cultured cell systems.

The next step—delivering the gene to the recipient cell—is being approached largely through the use of retroviral vectors. Here again, we are quite far along in "tailoring" vehicles which will safely and efficiently transfer a human gene into a recipient cell and enable it to be integrated into the genome. Unfortunately, we cannot yet control the site at which the gene will be integrated, but such control does not appear to be a necessary corollary to moving forward. A major current stumbling block, however, is at the next step, namely getting expression of the inserted gene in the recipient cell. For reasons still poorly understood, it has been very difficult to "turn on" the inserted gene after integrating it into the recipient cell's genome. In some instances the gene is expressed in cultured cells but not when the cells are returned to an experimental animal such as a mouse or monkey. In others, even expression in cultured cells has not yet been accomplished. Until this problem is unraveled, there is no likelihood of success and, therefore, no reason to perform a trial of gene therapy. In my view, it will take two to four more years before we know enough about controlling gene expression to bypass this block. Then, and only then, will we be in a position to implement such a strategy in man and monitor for its untoward as well as beneficial effects. I have watched the evolution of this field and have been reassured by the enormous care and rigor of most investigators who are trying to make human gene therapy a reality. They have worked in an atmosphere both open and critical. They have subjected themselves to ethical scrutiny throughout. That bodes well for the future of this potentially significant modality.

Prevention

The predictive power of genetics has been and will always be one of its major features. Because we know what genes are, how they work, and how they are inherited, we can tell family members whether they are or are not at risk for any given genetic disorder. For multifactorial traits and most chromosomal defects, such predictions are based on empiric risk data; for single gene defects, prediction follows Mendelian law of inheritance. Not surprisingly, therefore, disease prevention has been the "long suit" of clinical genetics to date. Preventive strategies have been both primary (i.e., prevention of conception) or secondary (i.e., prevention of birth). For example, a man whose mother died of Huntington's disease and who knows, therefore, that he has a 50 percent chance of developing the disorder may decide either not to marry, or not to have any children, or not to have children conceived from his sperm. Any of these options constitutes primary prevention because the disorder will not be transmitted to the next generation. Mankind's desire to reproduce, however, is powerful; for this reason many people take risks—even as high as 50 percent—of having affected children.

For those individuals whose religious upbringing or moral scruples do not bar them from considering pregnancy termination, secondary prevention through prenatal diagnosis has become a major approach in the past fifteen years. Many disorders can now be detected early in pregnancy using visualization techniques or tissue sampling. In general, couples who use these techniques choose to terminate pregnancies in which the developing fetus is affected and to continue those in which the fetus is unaffected. In well over 95 percent of all instances, an unaffected fetus is found; thus prenatal diagnosis has permitted the birth of far more children than it has halted.

The kind of prevention we have discussed thus far involves individual families. But genetic risks also apply to groups; major differences occur among different racial or ethnic groups with regard to the incidences in them of a variety of conditions. Cystic fibrosis, for example, is almost never observed in blacks but is frighteningly common in Caucasians of North European extraction. Conversely, hemolytic anemia due to glucose-6-phosphate dehydrogenase deficiency occurs in 10 percent of black men but in much less than 1 percent of whites.

All of these issues have led to the development of a new discipline called genetic epidemiology which concerns itself with the importance of genetic factors in the risks that populations have for one condition or another. This field has been energized by the realization that the interaction between heredity and environment can be crucial in predicting whether a given individual will develop a disease and when. Let me provide an example of such gene-environment interaction or, as it has been called, ecogenetics. Individuals with severe deficiency of a circulating anti-protease called α_1-antitrypsin generally develop pulmonary emphysema by their forties and often die of respiratory failure in their sixties. If such individuals smoke cigarettes, however, their life expectancy is reduced by approximately twenty years. Clearly, prudence dictates that such individuals (who constitute 0.1 percent of our population) not smoke, but such counselling requires that they be identified. We can think of this as another level of prevention—tertiary prevention—in which a specific environmental risk factor is avoided by a person or group with a particular genetic predisposition.

The new genetics will have major effects on all three levels of prevention discussed above. When, for instance, gene probes specific for Huntington's disease are available, the man described earlier will be able to find out if he has the mutant gene and will not have to base his procreative decisions on probability. Thus, if he is affected and desires to have only unaffected children, his wife's pregnancies can be monitored. As the linkage map of the human genome becomes progressively filled in, DNA probes will be developed for an enormous array of diseases. It is difficult to overestimate the power of this approach because our daily newspapers tell us weekly of its power: manic-depressive illness described in the Amish one week[23]; familial Alzheimer's disease[24] reported in the next. Within five years, the entire human genome is likely to have markers regularly placed along its entire length; those markers will then constitute a library of reagents with which we can detect and prevent disease. The larger the fraction of the genome we map and the larger the repertoire of diagnostic probes, the greater the applicability of this approach for primary, secondary, and tertiary prevention. In fact, as U.S. medicine and society becomes more oriented toward health maintenance and disease prevention and less oriented toward crisis management and death forestalling, this new genetic technology will be appreciated for the revolutionary development it is.

Obstacles to Progress

I have just described a number of ways in which new genetic technologies and strategies may affect the future of clinical medicine. Clearly, such applications will occur at different rates depending on a number of variables beyond those of the science, per se. Some of these variables constitute real or potential obstacles and they deserve mention.

Public and Professional Ignorance

Only a small fraction of the lay public understands even the rudiments of biology. Furthermore, few can comprehend the principles of probability upon which so much of genetic counselling rests. Because mankind distrusts and fears that which he/she does not understand, this widespread ignorance is responsible, in part, for societal ambivalence toward scientific advances in genetics. To solve this serious problem, more information about biology—human biology, particularly—must find its way into the curriculum of our elementary and secondary schools. Only an informed public will benefit maximally from the potential applications of the new genetics.

Many physicians, nurses, and other allied health care personnel are as ignorant of the principles of genetics as is the lay public. This serious obstacle to progress reflects the fact that scientific progress in this field has occurred so rapidly that it has postdated the formal education of most health care professionals. This problem is, however, self-limiting since the current generation of doctors and other health workers are being educated about the field. Nonetheless, the two generations of practicing physicians whose education preceded the revolution in our understanding of human genetics are generally ill-prepared to discuss clinical medicine in genetic terms, and are sometimes defensive or dogmatic about the area as a result.

Ethical Dilemmas and Choices

As mentioned earlier, our society has become accustomed to debates concerning the ethics of advances in genetics. Such debates will and should continue, but they must be framed in such a way that the views of all concerned citizens are heard—not merely those of a vocal and passionate minority. I am as concerned about those who would propose to use gene therapy to enhance such complex traits as intelligence as I am about those who urge that all research aimed at making gene therapy a reality be prohibited. Both groups insist their views are educated by ethical insights. Too often, however, partisans mistake religion or class-based prejudice for ethical concerns. However deeply felt, for example, the Catholic Church's view on abortion may be, it must be only one voice heard in the debate on the use of prenatal diagnosis of genetic disorders. Similarly, those who advocate banning genetic screening in the workplace for fear that employers will misuse the information to discriminate against blacks or some other group must hear from others who point out that some individuals and groups have innate risk factors worth their considering when entering the job market. Only sustained and open dialogue will ensure that an enlightened, judicious view will prevail; geneticists and other biological scientists must be prepared to participate in such debates, regardless of the associated demands on time and energy.

Resource Allocation

Because rDNA technology is versatile, simple, and inexpensive, its applications meet the crucial criteria for "high" technology; this contrasts with most of the current halfway technologies of clinical medicine whose distinguishing features are great expense and limited efficacy. Therefore, it is being argued, the rate at which the new genetics will be applied to clinical medicine as well as the speed with which it will offer new insights into such basic biologic processes as evolution, development, and differentiation, depends to an unusually great degree on how much financial support is directed toward it. This is nowhere more obvious than in the current debate about mounting a major national effort to map and sequence the entire human genome. Proponents argue that this major achievement can be realized by the year 2000 if this country joins with Japan and Western Europe in investing large sums of money (perhaps a total of $3 billion) for the purpose. They contend that, without such a focused effort, it may take 100 years to reach the same goal. Opponents of the idea say that such a "big science" approach to biology and disease is unnecessary and will divert funds from traditional investigator-initiated research efforts which are making real progress toward understanding the genome of man and other animals. This debate is currently being conducted in committees assembled by the National Institutes of Health (NIH), the Department of Energy, the congressional Office of Technology and Assessment (OTA), the National Research Council (NRC) of the National Academy of Sciences, and by various international consortia. Its outcome will influence, in a major way, how and when new genetic technologies will reach the clinical arena.[25]

The Humbling of Physicians

Among the many upheavals taking place currently in the U.S. system of health care delivery, that concerned with a loss of respect for and credibility of physicians is particularly worrisome to me as a medical school dean. The upward spiral in health care costs, driven in part by a thoughtless and greedy rise in physicians' fees, has resulted, along with the increasingly visible evidence through malpractice claims that physicians make numerous errors in their practices, in widespread dissatisfaction of the lay public with physicians and in an equally major souring of physicians toward their career opportunities. This dangerous confrontation can be lessened if physicians reaffirm their primary allegiance to their patients and the public good rather than to their guild and private gain and if those in charge of federal and private health care financing understand that high quality medical care can be provided only with the leadership of physicians whose sensitivity, compassion, and altruism can be combined with scientific sophistication and inquisitiveness. These latter qualities will not be found in doctors harnessed to some cost-driven, managed health care scheme which places a premium on following some rote order of testing and treating. Failure to appreciate this will result in the worst possible scenario— namely that in which the bright and caring people who still fill our medical school classes will be replaced by students of lesser intellect and capacity to adapt to a rapidly changing biological and medical world. This baleful outcome would be a disaster, not only for applying the new genetics to clinical medicine, but also for our whole society committed as it is to the notion that good health and good medicine are among the unalienable rights of all our citizens.

Notes

1. L. E. Rosenberg, "New Genetics and Old Values," *Pharos* 46 (1983):13–19; and L. E. Rosenberg, "Can We Cure Genetics Disorders," in A. Milunsky and G. J. Annas (eds.), *Genetics and the Law* (New York: Plenum Press, 1985), pp. 5–13.

2. K. L. Woodward, R. Cohn, and K. Springen, "Rules for Making Babies," *Newsweek*, 23 March 1987, pp. 42–43.

3. President's Commission for the Study of Ethical Problems in Medicine and Biomedical and Behavioral Research, *Splicing Life: A Report on the Social and Ethical Issues of Genetic Engineering with Human Beings* (Washington, D.C.: GPO, November 1982); and Rosenberg, "New Genetics and Old Values."

4. B. J. Culliton, "The Academic-Industrial Complex," *Science* 216 (1982):960–962.

5. S. N. Cohen, "The Manipulation of Genes" *Scientific American* 233 (1975):24–33.

6. R. D. Hotchkiss, "Portents for a Genetic Engineering," *Journal of Heredity* 197 (1965):56.

7. D. E. Comings, "Prenatal Diagnosis and the 'New Genetics,'" *American Journal of Human Genetics* 32 (1980):453.

8. D. Botstein, R. L. White, M. Skolnick, and R. W. Davis, "Construction of a Genetic Linkage Map in Man Using Restriction Fragment Length Polymorphisms," *American Journal of Human Genetics* 32 (1980):314–331.

9. President's Commission, *Splicing Life.*

10. President's Commission, *Splicing Life.*

11. S. H. Orkin, S. E. Antonarakis, and H. H. Kazazian, "Polymorphism and Molecular Pathology of the Human Beta-Globin Gene," in E. B. Brown (ed.), *Progress in Hematology, XIII* (New York: Grune and Stratton, 1983), pp. 49–73.

12. D. J. Weatherall, *The New Genetics and Clinical Practice, Second Edition* (Oxford: Oxford University Press, 1985).

13. R. G. Knowlton et al., "A Polymorphic DNA Marker Linked to Cystic Fibrosis is Located on Chromosome 7," *Nature* 318 (1985):380–382.

14. L. M. Kunkel et al., "Specific Cloning of DNA Fragments Absent from the DNA of a Male Patient with an X Chromosome Deletion," *Proceedings of the National Academy of Sciences* 82 (1985):4778–4782; and A. P. Monaco et al., "Isolation of Candidate cDNAs for Portions of the Duchenne Muscular Dystrophy Gene," *Nature* 323 (1986):646–650.

15. J. F. Gusella et al., "A Polymorphic DNA Marker Genetically-Linked to Huntington's Chorea," *Nature* 306 (1983):234–238.

16. P. H. St. George-Hyslop et al., "The Genetic Defect Causing Familial Alzheimer's Disease Maps on Chromosome 21," *Science* 235 (1987):885–890.

17. M. Baron et al., "Genetic Linkage Between X-Chromosome Markers and Bipolar Affective Illness," *Nature* 326 (1987):289–292; and J. A. Egeland et al., "Bipolar Affective Disorders Linked to DNA Markers on Chromosome 11," *Nature* 325 (1987):783–787.

18. M. S. Brown and J. L. Goldstein, "A Receptor-Mediated Pathway for Cholesterol Homeostatis," *Science* 4 (1986):34–47

19. J. M. Bishop, "Viral Oncogenes," *Cell* 42 (1985):23–38; and R. A. Weinberg, "The Action of Oncogenes in the Cytoplasm and Nucleus," *Science* 230 (1985):770–776.

20. Weatherall, *The New Genetics and Clinical Practice.*

21. Weatherall, *The New Genetics and Clinical Practice.*

22. W. F. Anderson, "Prospects for Human Gene Therapy," *Science* 226 (1984):401–409; and Weatherall, *The New Genetics and Clinical Practice.*

23. Egeland et al., "Bipolar Affective Disorders."

24. St. George-Hyslop et al., "The Genetic Defect Causing Familial Alzheimer's Disease."

25. L. Thompson, "Genes, Politics and Money," *Health, The Washington Post,* 24 February 1987, pp. 14–16; and L. Thompson, "The Race is on to Map the Gene" *The Washington Post, National Weekly Edition,* 16 March 1987, pp. 11–12.

8

Themes and Policies

Eli Ginzberg

Rather than attempt a comprehensive summary of the foregoing chapters and the discussion they elicited, an impossible task, this concluding chapter will identify a number of common themes that were developed by many, if not all, of the authors and discussants and will delineate some of the implications for policy that flow from them. It should be read as an interpretative review and assessment rather than as a consensus statement representative of all of the participants.

- The inherent dilemma for access to health care that arises from the conflict of the pervasive inequality of income and racial discrimination in the United States, and the accepted religious, moral, and ethical imperative that every human being is entitled to receive essential care.

This dilemma has been complicated in recent years by the collision of the historic ethical commitment of the physician to spare no effort in his responsibility to his patient and a gathering consensus that the enormous costs of providing medical care must be controlled.

The issue of conflicting professional and societal values and objectives has been intensified by the fact that in the decade and a half following the passage of Medicare and Medicaid (1965–1980) the liberal flow of private and public funds reinforced the professional ethic by providing the means for the physician to do everything needed for the patient's benefit. Cost was no longer a factor in the decision-making calculus.

Few health care analysts are aware that over half of all the physicians who are now in practice began their professional careers after the establishment of Medicare and Medicaid, when the issue of cost restraint faded into insignificance. These physicians face a particular challenge now that constraint in resource use is again a priority. Unlike their older colleagues, particularly those now in their seventies whose professional experience dates to the pre-World War II era, the younger members are confronting an environment which many, perhaps most of them, have not previously encountered.

How will the tension between a constrained amount of resources and the physician's injunction to do all that is possible for his patient be resolved? A number of policy directions are likely. The principle of "optimal" treatment for all will need to be redefined as "essential" treatment for all. At the same time, specific efforts must be undertaken by the federal and state governments to improve Medicare (catastrophic insurance for acute care has already been proposed); to introduce less stringent eligibility criteria and procedures for enrollment in Medicaid (some states); to impose a surcharge on hospital admissions and/or bills for redistribution to hospitals that provide large amounts of uncompensated care (some states); and to experiment with subsidized insurance programs for small groups/high-risk persons without coverage (some states). In addition, intensified efforts by the insurance sector are needed to develop coverage for long-term care (just beginning).

In the event that such efforts fail to stem the trend of ever larger numbers of persons lacking adequate health care coverage, the re-emergence of a national health insurance program on the nation's legislative agenda is a distinct possibility.

- A closely related theme is the tension between a constantly expanding technology and the narrowing margins for effectiveness in an increasing aged population.

Medicine is characterized by uncertainty with respect to diagnosis, therapy, and outcome. The most skilled physician can never be sure that the treatment that he recommends will yield a net benefit to the patient in terms of relief from pain, amelioration, or cure. As more and more people reach their eighties and nineties, their potential years of life are inevitably few in comparison to patients who are young or middle aged. Many, though not all, of the elderly suffer from one or more chronic ailments for which medicine has no cure; at best it can provide palliation. And further, many of those suffering from chronic illness can no longer care for themselves without assistance and in some cases, around-the-clock attention.

In the face of these narrowing margins for effective intervention, the question arises as to whether the full panoply of high-tech medicine, such as organ transplantation, open heart surgery, and other costly procedures, should be made available to all without regard to age.

Similar uncertainty attends the decision to initiate or discontinue life-prolonging treatment in the case of the severely ill, many of whom are, or may soon be, terminal. A disproportionate amount of costly medical resources is consumed by patients during their final year of life, in particular during the three months prior to death. The medical profession, however, is not well positioned to make a prospective judgment about who will live and who will die before initiating an expensive course of treatment. Faced with this dilemma, physicians are understandably loath to withhold sophisticated treatment until it is beyond doubt that the patient will never again become an independent, functioning individual.

But this is not the end of the dilemma. Some patients will opt to have their lives extended even if they will be bedridden to the end. And in a growing number of cases the patient is not capable of deciding and his relatives may be uncertain of his wishes.

It is evident that the advances in medical intervention, particularly those capable of prolonging life but incapable of restoring functionality, are precipitating unprecedented medical/social/ethical issues whose resolution will require intensive joint efforts of the public and the medical profession. Traditional approaches that were developed before the advent of high-tech medicine are no longer appropriate. However, the formulation of new guidelines for decisions that determine unequivocally the life or death of the individual require the utmost caution. Medical decision-making has become too complex and too far-reaching to be left to the judgment of physicians alone. The need to involve the patient in the decision-making process is compelling over the entire range of medical care, for it is the patient who must weigh the benefits and costs of alternative courses, guided by the information that his physician can provide.

- Another dimension of the changing parameters of health care delivery in a world in which medical knowledge and medical technology have become increasingly sophisticated and potent is the capacity of the medical profession to police itself and ensure that patients will not be subjected to harmful or worthless treatment.

In a litigious society, such as ours, a physician who is denied hospital privileges or whose license has been rescinded is likely to sue his peers for substantial monetary damages. Therefore, a hospital staff, a professional review organization, a county or state medical society, or a specialty group exercises extreme caution in bringing charges against a colleague. It is acknowledged, however, both by the physician community and by the more sophisticated members of the public that the issue of substandard medicine extends well beyond the group, however small or large, of incompetent or impaired physicians. Ineffective medical interventions, according to some analysts, constitute as much as 25 percent of the treatments provided by all practicing physicians.

Consider: At any point in time, the profession is composed of as many as three different cohorts of physicians who differ in educational and technical background and in experience: recent graduates of residencies and fellowships, who are in their late twenties and thirties; those circa forty-five to fifty years of age who are well established with half a career back of them; and the oldest group, over fifty, who may continue in active practice for some ten to fifteen years but are then likely to retire or to reduce their working hours and perhaps limit the scope of their professional activities.

The major mechanism for assuring that these several cohorts practice the "best" medicine, informed by the latest knowledge and utilizing currently approved procedures and drugs, is an elaborate system of continuing education (informal and formal) via journal literature, staff conferences, professional meetings, courses, lectures, and demonstrations, etc. Many busy practitioners, however, devote less time than is required to keeping current in their field, and many are unaware of the differences between normative local and regional practices and the clinical practices of colleagues elsewhere.

The National Institutes of Health have, through "consensus conferences," sought to establish and popularize the "best" practice in some highly controversial areas, such as the differential indications for vaginal deliveries and caesarian sections, or the criteria for assigning patients with cardiovascular diseases to medical or surgical treatment.

The follow-up to the reports and recommendations of the consensus conferences suggests that they have had limited success in altering physician behavior in favor of the preferred practices. The more generic issues in improving medical practice relate to the difficulty of collecting the basic data required for outcome evaluation and of establishing a mechanism that will both disseminate the results and assure compliance with the recommendations, particularly those that indicate the reduction/elimination of procedures that are in wide use. It is easier to demonstrate that many current practices and procedures are equivocal or counterindicated than to develop the professional and societal mechanisms to eliminate them at a cost that would not exceed the gain. A feasible vehicle can be tightened institutional controls such as the proposed invigoration of the Joint Commission on Hospital Accreditation and the broadened evaluative efforts accompanying the growth of managed care delivery systems.

- A long unresolved issue is the conflict between the physician's responsibility to recommend to his patient the preferred course of

> treatment (which may, in fact, be to desist from treatment) and his economic self-interest in the practice of medicine. The issue cannot be defined simply as one of verified diagnosis and proven therapy. Many patients will be satisfied only if their physician pursues an active treatment program and their confidence in the physician often contributes to a favorable outcome regardless of the specificity of the treatment (the placebo effect). Given the uncertainty that attends any medical intervention, a physician who is under pressure from his patient may be inclined to initiate treatment rather than follow a more conservative course of watchful waiting. Moreover, a specialist is likely to be biased in favor of specialized procedures, since his judgment is influenced more by past successes than past failures.

The physician's objectivity in advising and treating patients is suspect of being compromised by the fact that he earns his living from the practice of his profession; this has led many countries to abandon the traditional fee-for-service system of reimbursement. But it is by no means certain that turning physicians into salaried employees solves the dilemma. There is considerable evidence that the conflict simply assumes a new form: many physicians reduce their hours of work, are less personally committed to their patients, or shift part of their energies to practice in the private market (Sweden, Israel).

Recognition that this conflict is inherent in the practice of medicine, at least as the health care system operates in the United States, and that it cannot be removed or resolved by shifting from a fee-for-service to a salary system should be a warning to decision-makers not to seek a simple resolution through legislative or regulatory changes.

A sure way of worsening the dilemma is regrettably the one that the United States followed in the 1960s—to expand by an order of magnitude the numbers of students admitted to medical school. Within fewer than two decades the annual output of graduates doubled. Although there is growing awareness inside and outside of the medical profession that the number of future physicians should be reduced (as well the number training to be specialists and subspecialists), the institutional barriers to taking such action remain. Even if the resistance were overcome and medical school admissions began to decline, it would be decades before the total supply would be significantly reduced. In the interim, it is inevitable that the steadily increasing number of physicians will explore ways to establish and enlarge their practices with consequent overtreatment of patients and an upward tilt of total health care expenditures.

- Physicians are understandably concerned about the growth of "bureaucratic medicine" and its consequences: the amount of time that they must devote to filling out forms; the many practices that prudence dictates they follow against the contingency of a malpractice suit; the rules and regulations that govern their use of hospital care for their patients; the length of time that they must wait to be reimbursed; the many demands by third parties to justify their charges; and numerous other interventions by outsiders between them and their patients which are dysfunctional to both patient and physician.

These concerns and complaints cannot be dismissed as the intemperate responses of a pampered profession long accustomed to having its own way. When, as a leading West Coast internist has reported, it is necessary to practice defensive medicine that adds some 15-20 percent to the cost of providing effective medical care, the incremental bill for the country as a whole approximates $100 billion (1987)! The restiveness of the medical profession with the growing "bureaucracy" should be a cause of concern not only to physicians but to politicians and the American people.

There is, however, another side to the coin. In 1950, the total health care expenditures of the United States amounted to less than $13 billion; the estimated figure for 1987 is $511 billion. Stated as a percentage of gross national product, this represented a rise from 4.4 percent to 11.4 percent, or 2.5-fold. Even after correcting for the substantial increase in the population (and its aging) and the decline in the value of the dollar, the outlays per capita increased even more—almost threefold.

Most of the new money to finance this rapid growth has been provided by government (all sectors), which now covers about 40 percent of the total, and insurance (mostly from employers) whose share comes close to 30 percent. With these two funders putting up together some $350 billion, it is inevitable that they should demand a prominent role in determining the volume and scope of services to be offered and the conditions under which they are provided. In our society, payers have a major part in shaping and reshaping the market.

Physicians must recognize and respond to the new reality that these two principal financers, together with the public, will have a greater voice in all decision-making that affects the magnitude of total health care expenditures. The challenge to the medical profession is to form an alliance with the public so that in a cost containment environment, the amount of dollar outlays will not be determined without regard for the quality of care.

- The final theme that emerged both in the contributed papers and in the discussions can be subsumed under the rubric of the "medicalization" of societal issues.

Seeking care from a physician often reflects the patient's need for emotional reassurance, for guidance in his present or future behavior, for counseling with respect to personal, familial, or business problems. In earlier generations, the individual was likely to consult his minister, priest, or rabbi for reassurance and advice but the secularization of the modern world, particularly in the more affluent countries, has replaced the man of the cloth with the physician.

Other societal forces also contribute to the trend to medicalization. The physician is held in high esteem; his capacity to diagnose and treat is viewed as a public good and our democratic value system has led to a consensus that all citizens must have access to a physician, particularly when they will benefit from essential health care.

Many disadvantaged persons who suffer from lack of education, adequate income, a job, family, racism, and, more recently, even lack of housing, and others who have run afoul of the criminal justice system may be classified and treated by the medical system since they characteristically have some physical, mental, or emotional pathology. But just as often their defects have other roots, such as poverty, isolation, frailty.

Our society is more disposed to helping the ill and tolerating aberrant behavior which has a physical or mental origin than it is to dealing compassionately with individuals who violate its laws and norms. A young man who sought to murder the President of the United States, once he was judged to be insane, was not subjected to the full rigors of the legal system. He was confined, instead, to a mental hospital and if sometime in the future he should be adjudged to be sane, he may be discharged.

The overlapping of health and social causes of ineffectiveness is nowhere more evident and mutually reinforcing than in the case of the elderly. Many of the aged suffer from chronic illness, from increasing frailty, from deteriorating mental faculties, but they are also weakened by their loss of family and social supports and these two sets of forces often cannot be distinguished. All that can be stated unequivocally is that the problems of incapacity among the elderly do not stem solely or even primarily from the deterioration of their health. The compounding of these two sources of ineffectiveness that is also found among criminals, drug addicts, alcoholics, and many adolescents is a warning that medicine needs to consider anew its appropriate role and limitations in seeking to deal with social pathology. Its role is evident in cases where defective health is a major component of the individual's malfunctioning. But medicine must be careful not to become the dumping ground for dealing with all of society's misfits, many of whom require a broad range of support services, from educational remediation to income. Unless medicine hews a clear line between what it can do effectively and the areas that lie beyond its competence, it runs the risk of becoming overextended. Society is then likely to downgrade its capabilities in the areas where it can perform with distinction. In that event, both medicine and society would be the losers.

The foregoing far from exhaust the themes that may be found in the contributed papers and the discussions that they elicited. But they do reflect a number of the generic issues in the domain of clinical decision-making and societal values. The purpose of identifying and elaborating on a limited number was to help the reader recognize that both medicine and society are entering a new era of interdependence. As new issues move to the top of the agenda, new answers require exploration and resolution. Neither will come easily or quickly. But their pursuit cannot be long delayed without danger to both the future of medicine and the society of which it is a subsidiary system.

About the Contributors

Robert H. Binstock, Ph.D., is Henry R. Luce Professor of Aging, Health, and Society at Case Western Reserve University. A former President of the Gerontological Society of America, he has served as chairman and member of a number of advisory panels to the U.S. government.

Robert H. Brook, M.D., Sc.D., is Chief of the Division of Geriatrics, Department of Medicine, UCLA; Professor, School of Public Health, UCLA; and Deputy Health Program Director, Rand Corporation. He is a former Carnegie-Commonwealth Clinical Scholar, Johns Hopkins.

Robert H. Ebert, M.D., D. Phil., is Special Advisor to the President, The Robert Wood Johnson Foundation; former president, Milbank Memorial Fund; Dean Emeritus, Harvard Medical School; and recipient of the Abraham Flexner Award for Distinguished Service to Medical Education.

Roger W. Evans, Ph.D., is Senior Research Scientist, Battelle Human Affairs Research Centers; Clinical Assistant Professor, University of Washington; and on the Board of Directors, United Network for Organ Sharing.

Eli Ginzberg, Ph.D., is Director of Conservation of Human Resources; Hepburn Professor Emeritus of Economics at the Graduate School of Business; and Director of the Revson Fellows Program, all at Columbia University.

J.G.G. Ledingham, M.A., D.M., F.R.C.P. is May Reader in Clinical Medicine, University of Oxford; Honorary Consultant Physician, Oxford Area Health Authority; and former Director of Clinical Studies, University of Oxford.

Leon E. Rosenberg, M.D., is Dean and Long Professor of Human Genetics, School of Medicine, Yale University; and member of the National Research Council Committee on Mapping and Sequencing the Human Genome.

John W. Rowe, M.D., is Chief, Gerontology Division, Joint Department of Medicine, Beth Israel and Brigham and Women's Hospitals, and Director, Division on Aging, Harvard Medical School.

Albert L. Siu, M.D., M.S.P.H., is Assistant Professor of Medicine, UCLA; Health Services Researcher, Rand Corporation; Brookdale National Fellow; and a former Robert Wood Johnson Clinical Scholar, UCLA.

Cornell University Medical College Third Conference on Health Policy

Conference Organizers

Thomas H. Meikle, Jr., M.D.
The Stephen and Suzanne Weiss Dean
Cornell University Medical College

Michael J. Sniffen
Executive Director
Cornell Health Policy Program
Cornell University Medical College

Eli Ginzberg, Chair
Third Conference on Health Policy

Conference Participants

Reubin Andres, M.D.
Chief, Laboratory of Clinical Physiology & Clinical Director
Gerontology Research Center
National Institute on Aging

Robert H. Binstock, Ph.D.
Henry R. Luce Professor of Aging, Health, and Society
School of Medicine
Case Western Reserve University

Stanley J. Brody, M.D.
Professor of Physical Medicine and Rehabilitation
School of Medicine
University of Pennsylvania

Robert H. Brook, M.D., Sc.D.
Senior Staff Health Services Researcher
The Rand Corporation
Professor of Medicine and Public Health
UCLA Center for Health Sciences

Robert H. Ebert, M.D., D.Phil.
The Robert Wood Johnson Foundation

Leon Eisenberg, M.D.
Presley Professor of Social Medicine and Chairman
Department of Social Medicine and Health Policy
Harvard Medical School

Roger W. Evans, Ph.D.
Senior Research Scientist
Battelle Human Affairs Research Centers

Sander L. Gilman, Ph.D.
Professor of History in Psychiatry
Cornell University

Eli Ginzberg, Ph.D.
Director
Conservation of Human Resources
Columbia University

J. G. G. Ledingham, M.D.
Nuffield Department of Clinical Medicine
John Radcliffe Hospital
University of Oxford

Norman G. Levinsky, M.D.
Wade Professor and Chairman

Division of Medicine
School of Medicine
Boston University

John W. Littlefield, M.D.
Professor and Chairman
Department of Physiology
School of Medicine
Johns Hopkins University

Kenneth M. Ludmerer, M.D.
Associate Professor of Medicine
School of Medicine
Associate Professor of History
Faculty of Arts and Sciences
Washington University

Jerold Mande, M.P.H.
Legislative Assistant
U.S. Senate

Thomas H. Meikle, Jr., M.D.
The Stephen and Suzanne Weiss Dean
Cornell University Medical College

Arno G. Motulsky, M.D.
Professor of Medicine and Genetics
Director, Center for Inherited Diseases
University of Washington

Thomas G. Pickering, M.D.
Associate Professor of Medicine
Cornell University Medical College

Fred Plum, M.D.
Professor and Chairman
Department of Neurology
Cornell University Medical College

John Robertson, J.D.
Baker and Botts' Professor
School of Law
University of Texas at Austin

Leon E. Rosenberg, M.D.
Dean
School of Medicine
Yale University

John W. Rowe, M.D.
Chief, Gerontology Division
Beth Israel and Brigham and Women's Hospitals
Director, Division of Aging
Harvard Medical School

Hirsch Ṡ. Ruchlin, Ph.D.
Professor of Economics in Public Health and Medicine
Cornell University Medical College

Stephen C. Scheidt, M.D.
Assistant Dean and Professor of Clinical Medicine
Cornell University Medical College

Robert Sigmond
Scholar in Residence
School of Business
Temple University

Albert L. Siu, M.D., M.S.P.H.
Health Services Researcher
The Rand Corporation
Assistant Professor of Medicine
UCLA School of Medicine

Jerome M. Ziegler, Dean
New York State College of Human Ecology
Cornell University

Index

Aaron, Henry, 50
Abortion, 118, 128
Acute myocardial infarction. *See* Myocardial infarction, acute
Acylstreptokinase, 56
Adenosine deaminase deficiency, 125
Aging and the elderly, 15, 22, 83, 133–134, 138
  and carbohydrate metabolism, 101–102
  cognitive function, 103–104
  concept of normality, 99–104
  costs of dying, 106–109
  functional capability, 105
  geriatric syndromes, 105
  health promotion and disease prevention, 104–105
  and osteoporosis, 102–103
  population characteristics, 96–98
  population trends, 4, 31, 85, 96
  rationing of health care, 105–110
  successful and usual processes, 4–5, 99–100, 105
  transitions in status, 104–105
AIDS, 9, 15, 18, 122
Alcohol consumption
  and hypertension, 39–40
  and osteoporosis, 102
Allied health and paramedical personnel, 52, 128
Alzheimer's disease, 97, 119, 127
Ambulance service, 52–53
Amish, 127
Amniocentesis, 16. *See also* Prenatal care and diagnosis
Anemia, 118, 123
Anencephaly, 116
Angina pectoris, 9, 45–51
Antibiotics, 8–9, 123
Anticoagulants, 55–56
Antihypertensive drugs, 34–37
Anti-insulin antibodies, 123
Artificial insemination, 16, 114
Artificial organs, 66
Asilomar Conference (1975), 116
Atrioventricular block, 56
Australia, 35, 41, 48
Australian National Blood Pressure Study, 36, 37(table)
Avery, O. T., 115

Baby Fae, 66
Beadle, G. W., 115
Belgium, 41
Berki, S.E., 76–78, 82
Beta-adrenergic blockade, 45, 53, 55(table), 56
Beta-globin gene, 118
Beta-thalassemia, 116, 118–119, 125
Biochemical individuality, 115
Biofeedback and relaxation techniques for hypertension, 40
Biomedical ethicists, 106
Biotechnology, 5, 114, 118
Birnbaum, H., 76
Birth control. *See* Contraceptives
Blacks, 4, 116, 126
Blood pressure. *See* Diastolic pressures
Body composition and the aging process, 100–102
Bone marrow transplantation, 25, 124
Botstein, D., 116
Boyer, H. W., 115
Bradycardia, 56
Braunwald, E., 46, 48
Bristol study (1976), 51
British Cardiac Society, 41, 43, 45, 52
Brown, M.S., 57, 120
Bulgaria, 35
Bureaucratic medicine, 137

CABG. *See* Coronary artery bypass grafting

Calabresi, G., 21
Calcium, 40, 45
California, 20, 26–27
Canada, 41
Canadian Air Force exercises, 40
Cancer, 9, 16, 108, 114
  genetic research, 120–121
Capitation. *See under* Reimbursement systems
Carbohydrate metabolism of the elderly, 101–102
Cardiopulmonary resuscitation, 52–53
Cardiovascular disease, 3, 10, 16
  morbidity and mortality rates, 35, 37, 44(fig.), 53, 55–57
  See also Coronary heart disease; Hypertension; Myocardial infarction
Carotid endarterectomy, 24, 28
CASS. *See* Coronary artery surgery study
Casscells, W., 24–25
Catastrophic illness, 62, 88–89
  defined, 76–78
  key elements and perspectives, 77(table), 78
Catholic Church, 114, 128
CBO. *See* U.S. Congressional Budget Office
Cerebrovascular disease, 29
Chemotherapeutic agents, 8
Children and adolescents, 10
Cholesterol, 3
Chromosonal defects, 117–118, 126. *See also* Genetics
Chronic disease, 9, 11, 97, 138
  conceptualization of costs, 80–82
  See also specific diseases
Cigarette smoking, 16
  and coronary disease, 40, 43–44, 98
  and hypertension, 35, 37
  and myocardial infarction, 49
  and osteoporosis, 102
Cloning, 115, 121, 125
Cognitive function and aging, 103–104
Cohen, S.N., 115
Colorado, 108
Colorectal cancer, 26
Columbia Presbyterian Medical Center (New York), 67
COMA. *See* Committee on Medical Aspects of Food Policy
Comings, D.E., 116
Committee on Medical Aspects of Food Policy (COMA), 41
Common Market Food Policy, 41
Communicable diseases, 8
Congenital heart lesions, 117
Contraceptives, 15–16, 18
Coronary angiography, 24, 51
Coronary artery bypass grafting (CABG), 23, 28, 49
  and angioplasty compared, 51
  frequency and cost, 24, 46, 48, 50
Coronary artery disease (CAD)
  diagnosis and treatment, 9–10
  morbidity or mortality, 35
  prevention, 40–45
  See also Coronary heart disease
Coronary artery surgery study (CASS), 45, 47(fig.), 48(table), 57
Coronary care unit management, 53, 55–56
Coronary heart disease, 8, 35, 42, 70, 98, 120
  death rates, 48–49, 63
  therapies, 43–45
  See also Coronary artery disease
Cost containment. *See* Health care economics, cost containment
Cost sharing. *See under* Reimbursement systems
Crick, F.H.C., 115
Cryobiology, 66
Culyer, A.J., 86
Cystic fibrosis, 114, 117, 119, 124, 126
Czechoslovakia, 35

Danish Society of Cardiology, 53
Danish Society of Internal Medicine, 53
Death and dying
  causes and risks, 81(table), 84(table)
  cost, 70–71, 106–109
  and hypertension, 37–38
  life prolongation, 80, 85, 134
Denmark, 53, 54(table), 55–56
Deoxyribonucleic acid (DNA), 115, 117, 119, 121–122, 127. *See also* Recombinant DNA
DHHS. *See* U.S. Department of Health and Human Services
Diabetes mellitus, 66, 101, 117, 120, 123
Diagnosis-related groups (DRGs), 25, 30
Dialysis machine, 66. *See also* Kidney dialysis

Diastolic pressures, 35–38
Diet
  and the aging process, 100–102
  and coronary diseases, 40, 45
  and hypertension, 37, 39–40
  and myocardial infarction, 49
Dietary salt and hypertension, 39–40
"Diet of Reason: Sense and Nonsense in the Healthy Eating Debate" (Social Affairs Unit), 45
Diptheria, 8
Disease. *See* Chronic disease; Infectious disease
Doctors. *See* Physicians
Down's syndrome, 117
DRGs. *See* Diagnosis-related groups
Drug addiction and AIDS, 18
DuPont Company, 49
D vitamin and hypertension, 40
Dwarfism, 123
Dystocia, 9

Eastern Europe, 35, 41
Ecogenetics, 126
Ecology of disease, 7–12
Economic costs of disease and illness, 78, 79(table), 80, 87. *See also* Health care economics
Educational attainment of the elderly, 98
Effective care. *See* Essential care
Eggers, P. W., 71
End-Stage Renal Disease Program (ESRD), 61–62, 86
  patient costs and disability benefits, 87–88
  reimbursements, 71, 72(table)
England. *See* Great Britain
Environmental exposure and the aging process, 100
Epidemic disease, 9
Eschemic disease mortality rates, 44(fig.)
ESRD. *See* End-Stage Renal Disease Program
Essential care, 2, 26
  defined, 22–23, 25
Ethics. *See* Medical ethics
Etiology and genetics, 117–121
Europe, 48. *See also* Eastern Europe; Western Europe
European coronary surgery study, 45–46, 47(fig.)
Exercise
  and the aging process, 100–102
  and cardiovascular disease, 40, 49
  and osteoporosis, 102
Extracranial-intracranial artery bypass, 29

Fayerweather, P.H., 49
Fee-for-service. *See under* Reimbursement systems
Finland, 41
Forthofer, R.N., 76
Forward genetics, 119
Fragile X syndrome, 117
France, 10
Fuchs, V.R., 21
Funkenstein, D. H., 13

Ganglion-blocking drugs, 35
Garrod, A. E., 115
Gene therapy, 123–125
Genetic disease, defined, 117
Genetics, 114
  and cancer research, 120–121
  and diagnosis, 5–6, 121–122
  and disease prevention, 125–127
  and disease treatment, 5–6, 122–125
  ethical considerations, 5–6, 18, 128
  etiology and pathogenesis, 117–121
  forward and reverse strategies, 119
  historical perspective, 115–116
  impact on society, 116–117
  obstacles to progress, 127–130
Genome, 119, 125
  mapping, 116, 127, 129
Geriatric syndromes. *See under* Aging and the elderly
Germany, 10
Germ line gene therapy, 124
Glucose tolerance, 101
GNP. *See* Gross national product
Goldstein, J.L., 57, 120
Gonorrhea, 15
Graying of the population. *See* Aging and the elderly, population trends
Great Britain, 10, 13
  cardiopulmonary resuscitation training, 53
  coronary heart disease, 3–4, 35, 40–41, 43–45, 50, 52
  distrust of technological medicine, 50

health care funding, 50
hypertension, 35–36
Green, R.F., 103
Gross national product (GNP), percentage for health care, 13, 21, 137
Growth hormone, 123

Hampton, J.R., 52
HCP. *See* Hypertension Control Program
HDFP. *See* Hypertension Detection and Follow-Up Program
Health care allocation. *See* Health care resources, rationing
Health care economics, 2, 7–8, 129
for catastrophic illness, 76–77
components and conceptualization of cost, 12–13, 67–68, 70, 77(table), 78, 79(table), 80–83, 87
cost containment, 13, 17, 20, 25, 29, 105–106, 109–110, 137
and family income, 76–77
indigent care, 20, 22, 109
longitudinal data, 81–82
for organ transplantation, 4, 61–62, 67–68, 69–70(tables), 71–76
patient charges, 68, 70
as a percentage of GNP, 13, 21, 137
procedure costs, 67
program costs, 67
provider costs, 68
See also Health care resources; Reimbursement systems
Health care policy and preventive care, 61
Health care providers, 22, 27, 72. *See also* Health maintenance organizations; Hospitalization and hospitals; Physicians
Health care resources, 50, 61
access to essential care, 2, 17, 21–25, 132–133
and the elderly, 105–110
first-and-second-order determinations, 21–22
rationing, 2, 20–22, 25–31, 105–110, 128–129
"tragic choices," 21–22, 26, 31
See also Health care economics; Health care services;
Hospitalization and hospitals
Health care services, 7, 13, 17–18
abuses, 2–3, 20, 23–25, 28
clinical guidelines, 27–28
implications of an aging population, 96–97
societal values, 3–4
See also Health care resources
Health maintenance organizations (HMOs), 5, 25, 72
Heart transplantation, 61–62, 78, 86
artificial organs, 66
costs, 24–25, 70(table), 71–72
donor selection criteria, 64–65
organ preservation, 66
and preventive health care compared, 83
survival and quality of life, 73, 74–75(tables)
Hemodialysis, 24
Hemolytic anemia, 126
Hemophilia, 121, 123
Hepatic disease, 70
Herpes, 122
Hitler, Adolph, 116
HMOs. *See* Health maintenance organizations
Holland, 48
Hollenbeck, C.B., 102
Home care, 11, 51–52
Homosexuality and AIDS, 18
Hormones, genetic production of, 114, 122–123
Hospitalization and hospitals, 2, 9, 11–12, 16
abuses, 23–25
acute myocardial infarction care, 51–52
costs, 29, 80, 82
death during, 85
and the elderly, 97
See also Health care services
Hotchkiss, R.D., 115
Humana Hospital (Louisville), 66
Hungary, 35
Huntington's disease, 114, 119, 126–127
Hypercholesterolemia, 117, 120
Hypertension, 25, 27, 120
essential, 117
malignant, 3, 34–35
mild, 36–40, 57
severe, 3
therapy, 34–40
treatment in the elderly, 104
Hypertension Control Program (HCP), 40
Hypertension Detection and Follow-Up Program (HDFP), 35, 37–38
Hypolipidemic drugs, 45

Hypotension, 56
Hysterectomies, 26

Iatrogenic myocardial infarction, 51
Immunosuppressive drugs, 9, 73
Indigent patients, 20, 22, 109
Infants, 5, 9
  premature births and smoking, 16
  See also Prenatal care and diagnosis
  Infectious disease, 15, 122
  alterations in ecology of, 8–9
  conceptualization of costs, 80–81
  See also specific diseases
Inguinal hernia repair, 23
Institute of Medicine, 20
Insulin, 66, 101–102, 114, 123
Insurance companies and plans, 21–22
  cost containment interests, 105–106, 110
  cost sharing by consumers, 25–26
  organ transplantation coverage, 67–68, 72
In vitro fertilization, 114
Ireland, 41
Ischemic heart disease, 35, 37, 45
Israel, 136
Italy, 53, 101, 116

Jakob-Creutzfeldt disease, 123
Japan, 129
Jennett, B., 50
Jews, 116
Joint Commission on Hospital Accreditation, 135

Kaiser Permanente hospitals, 16
Kidney dialysis, 71
  machines, 66
  quality of life, 75(table)
Kidney transplantation, 63
  artificial organs, 66
  costs, 70(table), 71
  donor selection criteria, 64–65
  number performed 1973–1985, 73(table)
  organ preservation, 66
  survival and quality of life, 74–75(tables)
Kobrinski, E.J., 76

Law of inheritance, 115, 117, 119, 126
Life prolongation, 80, 84–85, 134
Lipid metabolism, 57
Lipid Research Clinics Primary Prevention Trial, 42
Liver transplantation, 25, 61–63, 78
  artificial organs, 66
  costs, 70(table), 72
  donor selection criteria, 64–65
  organ preservation, 66
  and preventive health care compared, 83
  survival and quality of life, 74–75(table)
LoGergo, J.P., 26
Loma Linda University Medical Center, 66
London Times, 18
Lubitz, J., 70, 107–108
Luft, H.S., 26

McCarth, 115
McLeod, 115
Madsen, E.B., 53
Manhattan project, 10
Manic-depressive illness, 119, 127
Maryland, 82
Matrix of medicine, 19
  defined, 7
  impact of science and technology, 11–14
  policy implications, 14–18
Matteson, A.L., 76
Mayo Clinic, 88
MCSSs. *See* Mechanical circulatory support systems
Measles, 8
Mechanical circulatory support systems (MCSSs), 66
Mechanical replacement organs. *See* Artificial organs
Medicaid, 2, 15, 20, 22–23, 27, 132–133
  cost containment interests, 109–110
  costs for the elderly, 105
Medi-Cal, 26–27
Medical economics. *See* Health care economics
Medical education, 7, 12, 17
Medical ethics, 106, 132–133
  and the new genetics, 128
  of organ transplantation, 4
Medical instruments, 10–12
Medicalization of social problems, 18–19, 138–139
Medical Research Council (MRC), hypertension study, 36, 38, 57
Medicare, 2, 15, 67–68, 132–133
  cost containment interests, 109–110
  coverage, 21–24, 70–71, 72(table), 105–109

Medicine, 1, 7–10, 14. *See also* Health care resources; Matrix of medicine
Men, 65
 coronary heart disease, 40–41, 42–43(figs.)
 ischemic disease, 44(fig.)
 osteoporosis, 102
Mendel, Gregor Johann, 115, 117, 119–120, 126
Menopause, 102
Mill, John Stuart, 41
Minorities, medical education, 14, 17. *See also* Blacks
Mitchell, J.R.A., 56
Mobile coronary care, 51–53
MONICA register, 50–51
Mortality rates, 38, 104
 from cardiovascular diseases, 35, 37, 44(fig.), 53, 55–57
 from myocardial infarction, 53, 55–56
 See also Death and dying
MRC. *See* Medical Research Council
MRFIT. *See* Multiple Risk Factor Intervention Trial
Multifactorial traits, 117–118, 126
Multiple Risk Factor Intervention Trial (MRFIT), 38
Muscular dystrophy, 117–119
Myocardial infarction, 10, 35–39, 41
 acute, 49(fig.), 51–52
 drug treatment, 53, 54–55(tables), 56

National Academy of Sciences, 129
National health insurance, 17, 87, 133
National Health Service (NHS) of Great Britain, 2, 50
National heart transplantation study, 65, 70, 74
National Institutes of Health (NIH), 10–11, 129, 135
National Kidney Dialysis and Kidney Transplantation Study, 74, 87
National Research Council (NRC), 129
National Task Force on Organ Transplantation, 72
Neonatology, 9
Netherlands, 41, 53
Neural tube defects, 117
New England, 23
New genetics, 115–116. *See also* Genetics
New Zealand, 35, 41, 48
NHS. *See* National Health Service of Great Britain
Nielsen, P.E., 53
NIH. *See* National Institutes of Health
Nitrate preparations, 45
Norway, 41
Nottingham team (1978), 51–52
NRC. *See* National Research Council
Nurses and the new genetics, 128
Nursing homes, 4, 97

Obesity and hypertension, 37, 39–40
Obstetrics, 9
O'Donnell, T.F., 70
Oncogenes, 114, 120. *See also* Cancer
One gene-one enzyme hypothesis, 115
Open heart surgery, 133
Oral hygiene and care, 98
Organ donors
 age criteria, 63, 65
 policies and legislation, 67
 supply factors, 62, 64, 65(table)
Organ preservation, 66
Organ transplantation, 9, 18, 78, 83, 88–89, 133
 costs, 4, 61–62, 67–68, 69–70(tables), 71–76
 ethics, 4
 need and supply, 4, 62–63, 64–65(tables), 66–67
 patient selection criteria, 63–64
 and preventive health care compared, 83
 survival and quality of life, 74–75(tables)
Oslo Study, 36–37
Osteoporosis, 97, 102–103
OTA. *See* U.S. Office of Technology and Assessment

Pancreas transplantation, estimated charges, 70(table)
Pathogenesis and genetics, 117–121
Patient charges. *See also* Health care economics
Payment methods. *See* Reimbursement systems
PCTA. *See* Percutaneous transluminal coronary angioplasties
Pell, S., 49
Penicillin, 8, 15, 34

Percutaneous transluminal coronary
angioplasties (PCTA), 48–49, 51
Peritoneal dialysis, 66
Peto, R., 43
Pharmaceutical drugs and industry, 8–12, 15, 73, 78
for cardiovascular disease, 34–39, 45, 53, 54–55(tables), 56
Phenylketonuria, 116, 121
Physicians, 2–3
bioscientific orientation, 13
career choice, 13–14, 17
clinical decision-making, 34, 106, 109, 135–136
education, 1, 135
ethical commitment, 132–133
excess of, 13–14
malpractice suits, 134–135
and the new genetics, 128–130
payment plans, 16–17
specialization, 11–12, 17
Plasma cholesterol concentrations, 41–43, 45
Plasmids, 115
Pneumococcal disease, 8, 34, 122
Poland, 35
Polio, 8
Polyunsaturated to saturated (PS) ratio, 41, 45
Post-infarction exercise ECG examinations, 56
Poverty among the aged, 15
Preferred provider organizations, 27, 72
Pregnancy and human behavior, 9
Premature birth and smoking, 16
Prenatal care and diagnosis, 18, 126, 128. *See also* Amniocentesis
Prepaid reimbursement. *See* Reimbursement systems, prepayment
Presidents, medical care for, 21, 88
President's Commission for the Study of Ethical Problems in Medicine and Biomedical and Behavioral Research, 117
Preventive health care, 5, 9, 89
and chronic disease, 83–85
and coronary artery disease, 10
cost effectiveness, 61, 83–85
for the elderly, 101–105
and genetics, 125–127
goal, 84
and life prolongation, 80
magnification of effect, 85
risks, 84–85
Prihoda, R., 70, 107–108
Procedure costs. *See under* Health care economics
Program costs. *See under* Health care economics
Prospective payment. *See under* Reimbursement systems
Proteins, production of, 122–123
Proto-oncogenes, 114
Prourokinase, 56
Provider costs. *See under* Health care economics
PS. *See* Polyunsaturated to saturated ratio
Pseudohypertension, 38, 40
Pulmonary emphysema, 126

Quality of life, 73, 74–75(tables), 76

Rand health insurance experiment, 23–25
Rationing. *See* Health care resources, rationing
rDNA. *See* Recombinant DNA
Recombinant DNA (rDNA), 5, 114
disease etiology, 120
and disease treatment, 122
and genetic disorders, 118
impact on society, 116
resource allocation, 128–129
technology, 115, 128–129
Recombinant human plasminogen activator, 56
Reimbursement systems, 16–17
capitation, 22
and choice of treatment, 34
cost sharing, 25–27
fee-for-service, 26, 29, 50, 136
preferred providers, 27, 72
prepayment, 26, 29–30
prospective payment, 22, 27, 29–30, 68
salary, 136
third-party payers, 24–25
Renal disease, 8, 71
Renal hemodialysis, 21
Research and the concept of normality, 99
Restriction fragment length polymorphisms (RFLPs), 116, 119

Retroviral vectors, 125
RFLPs. *See* Restriction fragment length polymorphisms
Rheumatoid arthritis, 26
Rockefeller Institute, 10
Rose, G., 57
Royal College of Physicians, 41, 52
Royal Society of Medicine, 53
Rubella, 8
Rumania, 35
Russell, L.B., 61

Salt restriction and hypertension, 39–40
Schaie, K.W., 103
Schizophrenia, 120
Schroeder, S.A., 76
Schwartz, W., 50
Science and technology, 12, 133
  and biomedical development, 10
  and the cost of medical care, 50
  and disease diagnosis, 121
  and disease ecology, 7–10
  follow-up and evaluation of new techniques, 29
  impact on the matrix of medicine, 11–12
  medical instruments, 10–12
  and the new genetics, 114
  new procedure development, 30–31
  of organ transplantation, 63
  and treatment choices, 34
Scitovsky, A. A., 106–108
Scotland, 41
Seattle, Washington, 52
Sentinel health events, defined, 30
Sexual revolution, 15
Sherry, S., 56
Sickle-cell anemia, 116–117, 125
Single gene defects, 117–118, 124, 126
Smoking. *See* Cigarette smoking
Social Affairs Unit (London), 45
Social costs of disease and illness, 78, 79(table), 80, 87. *See also* Health care economics
Social Darwinism and the valuing of human life, 86–87
Social Security, 15
Society
  and the matrix of medicine, 18–19
  medicalization, 6, 18–19, 138–139
  policy, 14–17
Streptokinase, 56
Stroke, 35–36, 38–39, 97
Surgical procedures, 11
  for angina pectoris, 45–46
  cost containment, 29
  geographic variations, 23
  international rate comparisons, 3
  rationing, 21
  second opinions, 26
  unclear indications, 23–24, 28
Sweden, 35–36, 41–42, 50, 53, 136
Syphilis, 8, 15

Tatum, E. L., 115
Tay-Sachs disease, 116
Technology. *See* Science and technology
Teenage pregnancy, 9, 18
Tetanus, 8
Thalassemias. *See* Beta-thalassemia
Thatcher, Margaret, 50
Thiaszide diuretics, 35
Third-party payers. *See under* Reimbursement systems
Thrombolytic therapy, 51, 56–57
Thrombotic cardiovascular disease, 123
Thurow, L.C., 29
Tobacco crops, subsidizing, 16
Tonsillectomy, 23
"Tragic Choices" (Calabresi and Bobbitt), 21
Transplant patients
  "ideal" candidates, 63–64
  quality of life, 74–75(tables)
  as risk takers, 83
  treatment, 62–63
  vocational rehabilitation, 73–74
Trisomy 13, 116
Tuberculosis, 8, 34
Turner syndrome, 117

United Kingdom. *See* Great Britain
United States
  coronary artery disease, 35, 41
  health care funding, 50
  hypertension, 35–36
  mobile coronary care, 52
Urea cycle disorders, 121
Urinary incontinence, 97
Urokinase, 56
U.S. Congressional Budget Office (CBO), 76
U.S. Department of Energy, 129

U.S. Department of Health and Human Services, 71
U.S. Food and Drug Administration, 16
U.S. Health Care Financing Administration, 71
U.S. Office of Technology and Assessment (OTA), 129
U.S. Surgeon General, 114
U.S. Veterans Administration (VA), coronary bypass studies, 46

VA. *See* U.S. Veterans Administration
Valuing human life, 85–89
Vatican, 114
Vectors, 115
Vegetarian diets and hypertension, 40
Ventricular fibrillation, 52
Verstraete, M., 56
Vietnam War, 14
Viruses, 115

Wales, 35, 41
Washington University Manual on Medical Therapeutics, 30
Watson, J.D., 115
Wechsler Adult Intelligence Scale, 103
Weight
  body composition and aging, 100–102
  and hypertension, 37, 39–40
Wennberg, J.E., 23
Western Europe, 3–4, 129
WHO. *See* World Health Organization
Willis, S., 103
Women, 65
  coronary heart disease, 40–41, 42–43(figs.), 98
  ischemic disease, 44(fig.)
  in medical school, 14
  mortality rates, 38
  osteoporosis, 102
  physician ratio, 17
World Health Organization (WHO), myocardial infarction registers, 49
World War I, 10
World War II, 8, 10–11, 22, 132

Xenografting, 66–67

Yarrow, Alfred, 41

Zavaroni, I., 101
Zook, C.J., 82